THE MANAGEMENT ANTHOLOGY SERIES

Edited by
Marlene G. Mayers, R.N., M.S., F.A.A.N.
Assistant Clinical Professor
University of California
San Francisco, California

Theme I.

The Organization: People and Structures

Organizational Theories and Structures
Organizational Units and Groups
Individuals in Organizations
Intraorganizational Conflict
Organizational Change

Theme II.

Management Functions

Communicating
Planning
Organizing
Staffing
Controlling
Leadership in Nursing

Theme III.

Product and Service Cost Effectiveness

Philosophy and Goals
Quality Measurement Methods
Maintaining Cost Effectiveness
Management Goals

Theme IV.

Employee Growth and Satisfaction

Motivation
Job Enrichment
Development Through Education
Development of Nurse Managers
Personal Growth

Theme V.

Organizational Security and Longevity

Organization-Environment Relationships
Social Policy and Nursing Services
The Women's Movement and Nursing
New Human Services and Technologies
Labor Relations in Nursing
Legal Protection of Patients and Nurses
The Politics of Nursing

Several volumes were in preparation when Leadership in Nursing
was published.

Leadership
in Nursing

Leadership in Nursing

Edited by

Marjorie Beyers, R.N., Ph.D.
Director
Evanston Hospital School of Nursing
Evanston, Illinois

The Management Anthology Series
Theme Two: Management Functions
Nursing Resources, Inc.

Nursing Resources, Inc.
12 Lakeside Park, 607 North Avenue
Wakefield, Massachusetts 01880

Introduction to the Management Anthology Series

As a nurse administrator or manager, have you often wished you could turn to your bookcase and select just the right book for the problem at hand? Or that you could talk with another nurse administrator who has faced a similar situation? Your time is limited, your problem is volatile, and the pressure merciless. Yet your bookcase contains no substantive reference source on current theories, thinking, or management methods.

Or if you are aspiring to become a nurse administrator or manager, do you wonder what you should read as part of your career development program? You may have scanned some management textbooks, only to find that, of necessity, they touch upon each subject briefly, leaving many questions unanswered and do not develop topics to any great depth.

If you are already a nursing manager or administrator or are planning to become a part of this challenging and important part of the nursing profession, you probably have discovered this problem; although there is a profusion of management applications available in the literature, they are scattered in a number of areas. And if you happen to stumble upon the application you need, it is not easy to relate it to a conceptual framework or to an overall philosophy of management. Thus you are left with a potpourri of articles and books that are as likely to be confusing as they are to be helpful.

The Management Anthology Series is designed to solve this problem by placing at your fingers a wealth of management information. Each book in the series focuses on one management topic;

each is an anthology—a collection of the best selections from the literature—about a specific topic. The selections are chosen by talented people, usually nurses, who are experts in a particular field of management. These editors have generously added their own wisdom, opinions, and nursing examples to the management literature, producing not just a compendium of articles, but a logical conceptual flow of current thought by the most respected experts on that subject.

The selections in each book are chosen to provide a specific progression of concepts, and each book, in turn, contributes to the overall conceptual framework of the series. Each article in each book is an integral part of a set of beliefs, goals, and content.

PREMISE STATEMENT   This series of books on nursing management is based on several premises. The interrelated components of this belief system illustrate the dynamics of the world of nursing administration and can be seen as a conceptual framework that ties each theme and each book into an understandable whole. The five major components, or themes, are:

1. The organization, its people, and its structures
2. Management functions
3. Products, services, and cost effectiveness
4. Employee growth and satisfaction
5. Organizational security and longevity

Theme 1: The Organization, Its People, and Its Structure

The organization is the basic social matrix of the conceptual framework because it contains the concrete interpersonal and intergroup processes through which social action is accomplished. Formal organizations require conscious and purposeful cooperation among people. As individuals, we recognize that cooperation is crucial; through it we can accomplish purposes that alone we are biologically unable to do. Cooperation is essential to the survival of an organization, and because cooperation depends upon communication and interaction, organizational units are usually limited in size.

Maintaining the fabric and patterns of cooperative enterprise is the job of managers, who are responsible for organizational structures, lines of accountability and authority, and individual and group responses to change. Theme 1, the organization as the basic social matrix of our conceptual model, is shown in Exhibit 1.

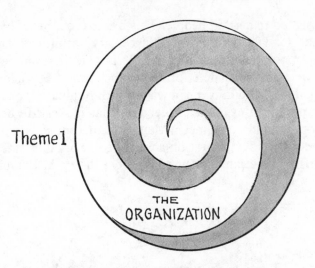

Theme 1

THE
ORGANIZATION

Exhibit 1.   The Organization, Its People, and Its Structure. (Theme 1.)

Theme 2: Management Functions

When Og, the prehistoric caveman, and his fellow tribespeople realized that they had to produce food to fill their hungry stomachs, they started communicating, planning, organizing, assigning jobs (staffing), and counting the cost (control and feedback). They also looked to someone to lead them. They didn't realize it, but they had to engage in management functions in order to achieve their goal—full stomachs!

Throughout the ages, this has been true of all collective human endeavor. Whether we realize it or not, we must fulfill management functions if we wish to achieve our goals. Seen in this way, management is not something forced upon people, it is a set of processes that we create for ourselves in order to ensure that we will be productive, satisfied, and secure.

The group initiates management tasks: communicating planning, organizing, staffing, controlling, and leading. These management functions are universal processes based upon a body of knowledge. When a group is small, the processes simple, and the products uncomplicated, each person may incorporate many elements of management into his or her day-to-day activities, such as patient care. As the group enlarges, as processes become more complex and specialized, and as products become harder to evaluate and count, the group designates certain people to do the jobs of management on behalf of the entire group.

In contemporary society, with its large corporations comprising thousands of people, various management functions have been assigned to certain people. This has led to a belief by some people that management is an unnecessary, arbitrary, and capricious group of people at the top. It is true in some situations that management has deteriorated to the level of capriciousness, but in most it is, and must be, a way of group thinking, planning, acting, communicating, and influencing that makes life better for both workers and consumers. Management functions arising from the needs of the organization and its people are illustrated as Theme 2 in the developing conceptual model shown in Exhibit 2.

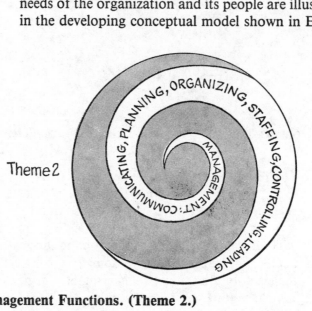

Exhibit 2.   Management Functions. (Theme 2.)

Theme 3: Product and Service Cost Effectiveness

People band together as an organization to produce something. Nurses come together to provide a service called nursing care, which is the profession's most obvious product.

An enterprise survives only so long as its "official," publicly of-fered products or services are marketable, or valued by society. Society expects an organization to produce products or services of quality at prices that are justifiable. To achieve this, nurse managers are responsible for defining values, formulating criteria, devising measurement methods, and setting forth, in under-standable terms, the quality and cost of nursing care services. Theme 3, product and service cost effectiveness, is shown in Ex-hibit 3 as one of nursing's outputs.

Theme 4: Employee Growth and Satisfaction

People want to grow and develop, and work enterprise has the potential for being one of society's most powerful instruments for

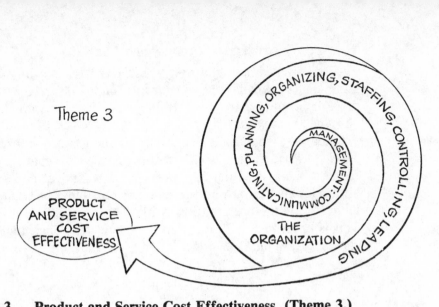

Theme 3

Exhibit 3.   Product and Service Cost Effectiveness. (Theme 3.)

individual growth. People are always "wanting and growing"; when one need is satisfied, another appears. This process is unending, continuing throughout one's life. Therefore, nurse managers provide for: a motivating environment, job enrichment, and educational opportunities for the group's members. An important organizational output is personal and professional growth and the satisfaction of its members. This component of the developing conceptual model is shown in Exhibit 4 as Theme 4.

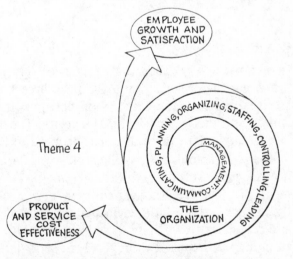

Theme 4

Exhibit 4.   Employee Growth and Satisfaction. (Theme 4.)

Theme 5: Organizational Security and Longevity

Finally, organizations must engage in transactions with both the internal and the external environments simply to survive, and even more importantly, to grow. If they cannot cope with their environments, they die.

Managers, who foster the quality of the group's transactions, develop sense organs to detect environmental changes. They forecast, plan, and develop strategies for survival and growth, always looking as far into the future as possible. The security and longevity of the organization is itself an organizational output. This is illustrated as Theme 5 in the completed conceptual model shown in Exhibit 5.

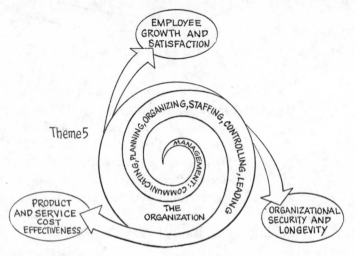

Exhibit 5. Conceptual Model for the Management Anthology Series. (Theme 5.)

Summary

In summary, this conceptual framework incorporates the belief that a nursing organization must have three major outputs: cost-effective patient care; satisfaction and growth for its members; and organizational security and longevity. The absence or diminution of any one of these three can jeopardize the others.

The conceptual model illustrates the organization of the Management Anthology Series. The major principles of management practice are interrelated in a comprehensive conceptual framework, whose basic elements are derived from the theories and principles set forth by such authors as Drucker, Odiorne, Etzioni, Benne, Bennis, McGregor, Herzberg, and Argyris. The conceptual framework is divided into five major organizing themes, each of which has multiple subtopics that are the focus of one or more of the resource books. Some subtopics of each of the major themes are listed in Exhibit 6.

Exhibit 6. Conceptual Framework for the Management Anthology Series.

Theme 1: **The Organization** includes books on:
Organizational theories and structures
Organizational units and groups
Individuals in organizations
Intraorganizational conflict
Organizational change

Theme 2: **Management Functions** includes books on:
Communicating
Planning
Organizing
Staffing
Controlling
Leadership in Nursing

Theme 3: **Product and Service Cost Effectiveness** includes books on:
Philosophy, goals, and criteria
Quality measurement
Maintaining Cost Effectiveness
Management goals

Theme 4: **Employee Growth and Satisfaction** includes books on:
Motivation
Job enrichment
Development through education
Development of nurse managers
Personal growth

Theme 5: **Organizational Security and Longevity** includes books on:
Organization/environment relationships
Social policy and nursing services
The women's movement and nursing
New human services and technologies
Labor relations in nursing
Legal protection of patients and nurses
The politics of nursing

Of course, any conceptual framework represents an arbitrary, yet defensible, division of content. The purpose of the division is to simplify a universe of knowledge so that one can grasp its essential nature. This accomplished, one can then deal with the myriad of details that logically (and sometimes arbitrarily) follow.

The conceptual framework of this series of books is designed specifically to provide nursing administrators and managers with current, comprehensive, and practical resources for dealing with management problems and issues. Each book relates to just one facet of management, and each selection covers theory as well as practical applications for nursing management situations, making it possible to review current thinking and practice quickly and efficiently.

Theme Two: Management Functions

There are certain activities that all managers perform. These functions are generic to management and necessary for any kind of organization to meet its objectives. Whether a group of people is producing cars, dairy products, safety pins, soap, or nursing care, management functions are universal processes that are based on a recognized body of knowledge. All administrators or managers must **communicate, plan, organize, staff, control** and **lead.** The proportion of time and energy spent on each of these functions varies widely from day to day, situation to situation, and from one level of management to another, however. The hierarchy of management roles determines which functions are most crucial at each level. Investigators have identified at least three different management levels: the institution, general management, and department management [1].

At the institutional level, the top executives (board of directors, chief executive officer, and so on) set overall objectives, assess the organization's environment, gather and allocate resources, and are accountable to stockholders or the public at large. Theirs is a trustee function. Top level managers make long-run, life-or-death organizational decisions rather than perform the daily operations work of the organization. Their major management functions are planning, controlling, communicating, and leading.

Persons at the next level, general management, are responsible for specifying the overall objectives, implementing action plans, and utilizing allocated resources to the best advantage. The functions crucial to these mana ers are communicating, planning, organizing, staffing, controlling, and leading.

Departmental level managers (department heads, first-line supervisors, and so on) are primarily concerned with on-line production. They must utilize people, money, and technology to coordinate the work flow and ensure that their departments contribute to the effective accomplishment of the organization's goals.

Not all organizations are large enough to provide for three discrete levels of management. However, every management or administrative group must fill these three levels of functions, either by incorporating two or three levels in one or more persons' roles or by changing focus from time to time.

Each of the series of books in this theme, Management Functions, attends to one of the tasks of a manager. These management functions represent the technology of management—the intellectual, physical, and psychological tools that administrators and managers must have at their disposal in order to carry out their work effectively.

This book is devoted to the leadership function of management. As the book defines and explains the meaning and skills of leadership, it becomes abundantly clear that the absence of effective leadership jeopardizes the success of all the other management functions.

References
1. Holden, P., Fish, L., and Smith, H. **Top Management Organization and Control.** New York: McGraw-Hill, 1975.

Foreword

Of all the management functions, leading or leadership is the most difficult to pinpoint. The other functions—planning, organizing, controlling, and staffing—tend to be more impersonal and could possibly be carried out by a manager alone in his or her office. But leadership is different. "It refers to the interpersonal process by which a manager seeks to influence employees to accomplish tasks. Leadership takes place not in isolation but in interaction" [1]. It is often said that leadership can more easily be recognized than described and is known more by its effects than its analysis. Of all the management functions, leadership probably has been the most studied, yet remains the least understood.

Barnard, in his classic book, **The Executive Function**, has described a leader as one who is influential, is confident, has a high level of vitality, and has a finely honed sense of judgment, proportion, balance, and timing. Barnard also characterizes a leader as one who is able to conceptualize the "big picture" and to communicate it to others.

Goble [2] says that leaders are not characterized by a list of personality traits designated by a leadership style. He believes that leaders "emerge from among those who best understand and are able to lead a society that will insist on" the following:

- An increasing emphasis on the quality of life rather than productivity or profit
- Interdependence rather than independence of groups and organizations

- Cooperation rather than competition
- More emphasis on social justice and equity and less emphasis on technological efficiency
- Development of an organization's people as individuals, rather than organizational convenience
- Participatory management
- Recognition of the work ethic as a means of self-enhancement rather than as a duty
- Leisure as a legitimate activity in its own right
- Incorruptible personal integrity and respect for the property of others
- More stress on personal responsibility rather than "let someone else do it"
- A clean and orderly society

How can one become such a leader? Is the quality of leadership associated with a position or title? Is it possible to be an effective leader in some situations and not in others? What types of leadership style are there? What are their pros and cons? How can a leader learn and act effectively in relation to society's values?

This book, edited by Marjorie Beyers, contains the best current literature on this challenging subject of leadership. Dr. Beyers has generously added her own perceptions and analyses to the subject in general and to the thoughts expressed by the many authors who have contributed to the book.

Marlene G. Mayers, R.N., M.S., F.A.A.N.
Series Editor

References
1. Hampton, D.R. **Contemporary Management.** New York: McGraw-Hill, 1977, p. 283.
2. Goble, R.L. Leadership in a society in transition. In Benton, L. (Ed.) **Management for the Future.** New York: McGraw-Hill, 1978, pp. 136, 137.

Acknowledgments

I wish to acknowledge Anthony Cresswell, Ph.D., Professor, and Carol Wolfe, Editor, for their ideas and assistance in preparing the manuscript.

Table of Contents

INTRODUCTION: A MODEL FOR LEADERSHIP

If I were to ask you to take me to your leader, who would that person be? Every one of us has a perception of leadership. Usually, our perceptions of leadership are results of relationships with people who have significant impact on our lives. How are the persons you identify as leaders different from others? Do those persons have innate characteristics that set them apart? Or are they leaders because of the way they have dealt with a particular set of experiences in a given social system? In this anthology we will explore some concepts and theories of leadership as well as some applications of these theories to leader-follower situations.

Although there are many theories about leadership, none provides an explicit definition of that term. It cannot be explained in the same way that one can explain how blood flows through the heart. The social systems of the world have always produced leaders. Over time those leaders have emerged from their groups of reference to give their names to inventions, to social phenomena, to political plans and doctrines, and to institutions. Leadership seems to be an essential part of life and the topic of leadership is relevant to many dimensions of group life. In nursing, leadership is important because nurses function within social systems. As a professional group, nurses are concerned with maintaining viable and productive leadership. This concern is complicated by the inability to clearly define or describe leadership through succinct application of theories and concepts.

From the outset, we should establish that leadership is not quantifiable. We do not know how best to develop leaders. We cannot always predict who will become leaders, but we know that nursing needs leaders to take responsive action in the field to solidify past accomplishments and to structure the future. We want leaders who will be "movers and shakers"—people who will bring about growth and change, who will make things happen. The nursing profession needs members who can exert a dynamic force in society.

We should also establish at the outset that leadership is important for every student of nursing. Most schools of nursing have as one of their objectives that graduates will become leaders. Is it possible for every single nurse to be a leader? If you consider that leadership is relative to particular situations, you might answer this question affirmatively. There are leaders in every group, but not always the same leaders. Some individuals who are followers in one group become leaders in others. In the nurse-patient relationship, every nurse is a leader.

In groups of nurses at every level in nursing, some individuals emerge as leaders of other nurses. When representing these groups at conferences or meetings these leaders form other groups. Some of those who are leaders "at home" become followers in the groups at the conference while some become leaders. Does all of this sound like double-talk? It is not meant to be ambiguous, but rather to clarify that leadership can be relative to groups or situations.

There are leaders at every level of nursing. One can find leaders among nurse aides, staff nurses, nursing administrators, and nursing educators. Although a person doesn't need a title to be a leader, leaders are often appointed to positions with titles like director of nursing, head nurse, or president. Because leadership is fluid the audience for this anthology can be drawn from any one group of nurses. It is practical to consider that everyone is at some time and in some place a leader. This anthology should be useful in many different contexts to help nurses formulate and develop their personal perceptions of leadership practice.

In order to bring some order to the complex subject of leadership, a model can be developed to illustrate how a nurse-leader functions. This model is based on the assumption that the behavior of individuals is a complex product of the interaction between the individual and the environment. Leaders are influenced by their environment and they also influence their environment.

In this model, we can consider that there are three major components of a nurse-leader's environment: the workplace, the profession, and one's personal life (Exhibit 1). The workplace can be any type of organization within the health care industry—a hospital or outpatient facility, an independent practice, an educational institution, an industrial health program, or a professional organization. The majority of nurses are employed by health care agencies of one type or another, and the exigencies of

the workplace influence the practice of nursing, just as nurses in practice influence the workplace.

Profession is another component of the leader's environment. The term profession has different meanings for different nurses. For the purposes of this model, we can define the nursing profession in the context of environment as an organized group that provides peer support and that is visible in society for clarifying and furthering the goals of nursing. The profession serves to perpetuate public sanction for its members; it expands and elaborates on the personal values, ideals, and practices of its members. The dynamic core of the professional groups of nurses organized to serve their members is the membership. The professional groups influence the members and members influence the groups. The result is a professional organization that has characteristics and attributes formed by the aggregate of members' behaviors. The phenomenon of organizational power thus formed supercedes that of any one member.

One's personal life is the third major component of the nurse-leader's environment. In this model, personal life comprises life-style, home, family, and community relationships. For some leaders in nursing, aspects of their personal lives have primary emphasis, whereas for others the workplace may take first place. Recent developments in definitions of the role of women in this country have brought attention to the fact that nurse-leaders, the majority of whom are women, can successfully combine commitments to professional and personal life. Nurses can be active family members and can have strong personal commitments. The nature of the leader's commitments to home, family, and community do have an impact on his or her commitment to and involvement with both the workplace and the profession in general.

It seems reasonable to assume that leaders in nursing must balance the amounts of energy they expend on each of their com-

Exhibit 1. Model for Leadership Behaviors

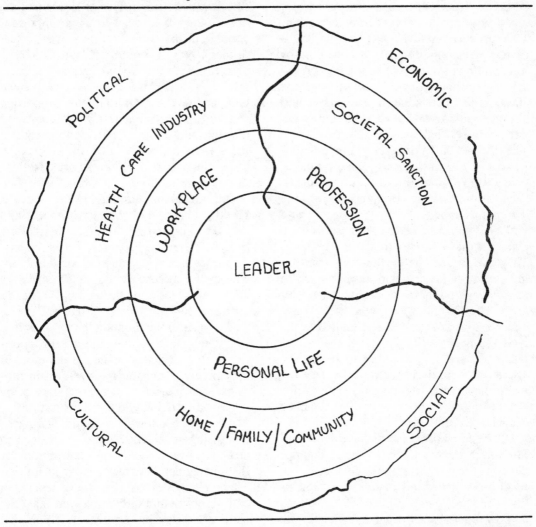

mitments in the three components of their environment. But the workplace, the profession, and personal life can also be a source of energy and inspiration for the leader. We might posit that successful leaders are those who can effectively balance the energies they expend on their commitments and actions in all three environmental components and benefit from the energy they receive from them. It might also be speculated that leaders are those who deal effectively with the peripheral components of our model—that

is, political, economic, cultural, and social aspects of the society in which they function.

That confusion exists about what constitutes leadership is shown by the diverse views of leadership presented in the selections you will read in this anthology. Several of the selections treat leadership and management as synonomous, implying that they represent similar aggregates of behavior. Not all leaders are managers, however, as indicated earlier. And the converse is true: not all managers are leaders. To elaborate this point let us consider that nurses practice within a particular structure of society, within a health care agency or another type of organization. This structure can be likened to a merry-go-round. We can envision the nurse-manager or leader riding the merry-go-round, always going up and down through the satisfactions and conflicts of leading or managing, and always moving through changing environments with different sets of events. The rider attends primarily to one environment at any given time and yet always maintains a fixed position through personal identity and through the integrating structure of the merry-go-round.

Nurses who are leaders and those who are managers have certain things in common. They differ perhaps in that the manager must perceive his or her position as tied to the merry-go-round—to riding a given horse. The leader however, need not perceive his or her position as fixed or limited to the merry-go-round's circular route, but can attain distances in any direction he or she selects. The terrain in the direction selected will in large part determine the type of difficulties or satisfactions, or both, that will be encountered on the leader's ride.

Differences between management and leadership are not clear. In many theories developed from research cited in the readings excerpted in this anthology, the individuals studied held management positions such as supervisor or department head. The theories may reveal more about how managers influence personnel to accomplish goals of an organization than about the influence of leaders. You may wish to consider every person in a management position as a leader. On the other hand, you may consider that some managers are leaders who perceive their environments differently. These leaders not only keep the organization running smoothly (a task of management) but also initiate change. Through innovation they improve the environments or the quality of work produced.

Throughout this anthology the relationship between the manager or leader and the organization is referred to as an important variable in the manager's or leader's effectiveness. Nurses should question their relationships with their organizations to determine how leadership and management can best be developed within the supporting structures of an organization. Nurses need not only to use the support and strength of these organizations, but also to make a perceptible impact on these organizations through the quality of their practice.

Our model implies that leaders have a broad perspective of their environment and that they successfully integrate the realities of the different environmental components. As leadership in nursing becomes increasingly influential the labels or titles assigned to positions nurses hold in health care agencies are changing. How a nurse-leader fits into the situation in the workplace is tantamount to defining that person's position in the workplace. The development of new titles for nursing managers in institutions is an indication that nurses are being perceived differently in those institutions.

In many hospitals, the traditional director of nursing service title is being changed to vice-president for nursing, chairperson for the nursing department, or other such titles. These new titles imply management roles and responsibilities that may or may not have been carried out by the traditional director of nursing service. Although the newer titles are sometimes merely word changes without accompanying role changes, ideally they should reflect the leadership exercised by nursing administrators or managers in the health care agencies. This anthology will establish the distinctions between actual leadership roles and management roles with only titular leadership in the organization structures of health care agencies.

Titles of other nursing personnel in health care agencies are also being changed. The traditional title "supervisor" is not universally used as it was in the past. In current practice one can find coordinators or managers functioning at the positional level formerly held by the supervisor. Team leader, staff nurse, and other such traditional titles are being replaced with the titles primary nurse, nurse clinician, and nurse specialist. These changes indicate increasing emphasis on the professional status of nurses in health care agencies rather than on the superior-subordinate relationships common to traditional and bureaucratic organizational structures.

Leaders in nursing are not just those people who have supervisory or management titles in the workplace. In this respect too management and leadership may be distinct. Leaders can be found throughout the ranks of nursing: among nurses' aides, licensed practical nurses, registered nurses, nurses with masters degrees and doctoral degrees, and nurses in the various fields of specialty practice, such as critical care. Each group of nurses has its leaders who strive to develop and to protect members' interests. This phenomenon suggests that leadership is a function of a social group, and that certain persons do have either innate or learned abilities to become leaders. Why do certain persons demonstrate the ability to influence others? Since leadership is displayed by members of every level of nursing, it is not necessarily dependent on educational preparation. Why then do group members perceive that a certain person is their leader?

Nursing professionals are expected to become leaders; it can be inferred from this belief that leadership can be learned. As a professional nurse, one is expected to be a leader in many activities: in giving patient care, in personal growth as a professional, in developing paraprofessionals through leadership in patient care, in community and professional activities that promote both the development of nursing and the health of the citizens. We must ask, is every nurse a leader by virtue of being a professional? Is leadership an aspect of the professional nursing role?

In the workplace, some nurses emerge as leaders; a few of these workplace leaders also emerge as leaders in the profession in general. Who are the nurses who emerge as leaders in the profession? Are these persons "superleaders"? We can posit that every professional nurse is a leader in some aspect of his or her environment as defined in our model. We can also posit that any definition of leadership can have varied applications. Because of the many facets of leadership, the term can be applied to a large number of different contexts, resulting in loose definitions and complexities in studying leadership.

One way of viewing leadership is from the context of a person's involvement in the three components of the environment. A nurse-leader who is actively involved in all three components of the environment, is exchanging ideas with other nurses in the professional component, in the workplace component, and in one's personal life. This individual can then integrate events in all three components, bringing professional issues and concerns into the workplace, and workplace issues into the professional component, and community issues into both of the other two. The stimuli occurring in all environmental components can be catalysts in promoting open communication, in identifying and solving problems, in clarifying values, and in bringing about change. To cross-fertilize the components in the environment one must be a well-integrated person who can balance the various components effectively.

Why is it necessary to balance environmental components? We have all known singularly dedicated nurses who give excellent patient care but who do not belong to a professional nursing group and do not know about current professional issues. We may also know nurses who work diligently to further the profession through employment in professional nursing organizations but who cannot relate to nursing practice in the workplace in any practical manner. We also know nurses who are equally involved in workplace, profession, and personal life. It seems plausible that the integrity of the professional organization depends on pursuing goals that are realistic in terms of actual nursing practice and of societal needs for nursing care. Similarly, the integrity of professional nursing depends on realistic striving for professional goals that strengthen and improve actual nursing practice. Thus, the effective leaders have greater impact or strength because they work toward achievement of goals that are congruent with those of persons in nursing's professional organizations and with the citizens in the community.

The nurse-leader's ability to balance the environmental components of his or her world seems to be a crucial issue in nursing today. As we further refine our model, we can understand that the balancing requires juggling opposing forces. In the social sciences, such terms as social pressures, conflict, stress, and social deviance are used to discuss problems of balancing the needs of individuals and groups in society with those of the society at large. The nurse-leader's environment is no exception to social interrelationships in general. Nurses are part of the broader health care industry which is currently undergoing close public scrutiny. The entire industry is changing in response to societal forces. Nursing, as one part of the industry, is greatly affected by events taking place in the entire industry.

There are many levels of conflict within the health care industry and within nursing specifically. Health care organizations have specific organizational goals and objectives;

goals and objectives that may be in conflict with those of varying health professional groups, with one's personal goals and objectives, or with societal needs. Conflict, then, is a realistic aspect of the leader's integrating of environmental components. Positive interaction skills, conflict resolution, and negotiation skills consequently become important behaviors for leaders in the model we are developing. How the leader interacts, resolves conflict, and negotiates is influenced by personal and organizational value systems, by perception of professional roles, and by skills one learns in the course of one's professional education and subsequent career.

The study of leadership is important to professionals, and leadership roles are relative to a person's environment as defined in our model. The emphasis of this anthology is on leadership for actively employed professional nurses. For this reason, most of the selections focus on relationships of people in the context of organizational behavior. Each reader will approach the study of these selections from an individual perspective and can derive personal implications from the theories and concepts presented. The model presented in these introductory pages is given as a matrix that can be filled in by the individual reader. The application of leadership theories to develop leadership skills and abilities has implications for all nurses.

Articles selected for this anthology are arranged in three units: 1) Leadership: Theories, Definitions, and Styles; 2) The Leader; and 3) Leadership in Organizations. Content about the behaviors of leaders is threaded through each of the selections in these three units even though the focus of a particular unit is slightly different.

UNIT 1 LEADERSHIP: THEORIES, DEFINITIONS, AND STYLES

The first selection of this unit is an excerpt of a chapter entitled "Leadership and Power" in a book written by Fred Luthans.† This scholarly overview of the classical theories of leadership may help you establish your frame of reference about leadership. The author presents these theories in the order of their development, demonstrating how the theories of leadership have evolved from the time of the Lippitt and White studies concerned with leadership styles to the recently developed path-goal theory of leadership.

In Luthans' essay, you are introduced to terminology used in discussing leadership as well as to the salient issues in research about leadership. It is a nice beginning point from which to fill in the matrix of our model since it contains sufficient information about each theory in a practical context. You can use this material as an introduction leading to further, in-depth study of leadership theories or to refresh your knowledge of leadership.

The issues raised in the article can be related to our introductory model because they focus on the leader's personal traits and characteristics, leadership in situations such as occur in all aspects of the environmental components of the model, leaders' effectiveness as described by Fiedler's contingency model, and the impact of leaders' behaviors on others as described by the path-goal theory.

The next two selections in this unit present theories of leadership as applied in particular ways. You will note that both authors refer to a theoretical framework of leadership. These frameworks have been developed from research findings or theories of leadership presented in Luthans' chapter. Each author elaborates on the

---

†In adapting previously published literature, the editor has added original commentary. Throughout the rest of this book, the editor's comments are italicized to distinguish them from reprinted material.

selected theories in a different way in applying the theories to practice. The articles demonstrate how theories can be "popularized" to become commonly held ideas about leadership. Pure theory can be adapted in application. The theory becomes less important than its usefulness in helping one to analyze and interpret events that take place when leadership is exercised. When one is responsible for working with others to accomplish work and to provide services, pure leadership theories seem less practical than adapting the theories to behaviors that provide direction for others. You may develop your own adaptations of leadership theories as you study the thoughts of others who are involved in explaining their perspective of leadership.

Heimann's article gives several definitions of leadership. It also presents leadership from the perspectives of traits, styles, and situation, and a synthesis theory termed the interaction theory of leadership. This article is useful because the author presents leadership in the context of nursing. Several points made by Heimann are worth noting: group leadership is fluid; the total culture from which a group emerges is one of the elements to be considered in situational leadership theories; the leader's position is changed by the forces in the field of the leader's position. Like our introductory model this treatment demonstrates dynamic interaction. Heimann's article illustrates that change is ever present and that leadership shifts according to changes taking place in one's environment.

Some authors in nursing have stated that the differences in role perception among nurses and within the health care industry are sources of conflict for professional nursing. When reading Heimann's article, consider how changes in the situations of the workplace, the profession, and your personal life can affect you in your capacity as leader. An awareness of the interaction among events is very helpful for determining how to evaluate change, how to control change for the benefit of the profession, and how to bring about change.

Appelbaum's article focuses on leaders' behaviors in the specific environment of one hospital. The study of relationships between leaders and followers in this hospital demonstrates how theoretical assumptions can be applied in an organization to produce leaders who are also managers. The capabilities of the leader for development of followers, for unifying them, and for supporting the goals of the organization are discussed from a theoretical viewpoint. The study is based on assumptions generated by research, including McGregor's Theory X, Theory Y theory and findings of the Ohio State studies. Comparing Appelbaum's emphasis on leader and follower behaviors with Heimann's focus on shifting situations and conflict can contribute to one's perspective on how management and leadership can be associated in attaining organizational goals

This comparison will also give insight into how cognitive dissonance about the expectations of the nurse's role can lead to conflict between the goals and objectives of the workplace and those of the profession.

The final article in this unit presents a systematic approach to leadership selection. The author, L. Plaszczynski, associates leadership and management and indicates how one organization uses common leadership behaviors to select leaders in different types of organizational positions. Consider this article in relation to theories of leadership. Are there differences between leading an autonomous professional staff and leading a staff comprised of paraprofessionals? In current nursing practice, the mix of types of nursing personnel with different levels of education and experience varies from one health care agency to another. Must each environment be analyzed for situational differences that arise from staffing pattern variations, the type of organizational structure, and the needs of group members? Or is leadership universal regardless of the situation?

This article is useful for exploring the implications of using a systematic approach to leadership selection. Does this approach allow for different types of leadership styles? Can an individual who has been an effective leader in one organization adapt his or her leadership style to the demands of a different organization? Or should the individual's leadership style be matched to a given organization? Is the selection process described in this article specific to the organization described? Does the selection panel personalize the selection process for the organization?

A pertinent question that emerges from the leadership selection process is: how much does one's personal leadership style or expectations of leadership roles influence one's potential for being successful in a given position? Consider that you are an applicant for one of the positions in the organization described in this article. What data would you assemble about the organizational structure, the staffing patterns, and the group members when making your decision about whether to accept the leadership position? Can you adapt and accommodate your personal leadership behaviors to the expectations of persons in this organization effectively? Or, if you are already a leader, will you be effective in any type of organization?

LEADERSHIP AND POWER
(an excerpt)

By Fred Luthans

THE BACKGROUND AND CLASSIC STUDIES ON LEADERSHIP

Leadership has probably been written about, formally researched, and informally discussed more than any other single topic. Throughout history, it has been recognized that the difference between success and failure, whether in a war, a business, a protest movement, or a basketball game, can be largely attributed to leadership.† Yet, despite all the attention given to it and its recognized importance, leadership still remains pretty much of a "black box" or unexplainable concept. It is known to exist and to have a tremendous influence on human performance, but its inner workings and specific dimensions cannot be precisely spelled out. Despite these inherent difficulties, a review of some of the widely known classic studies on leadership can help set the stage for the analysis of modern theories and styles of leadership.

Lippitt and White Leadership Studies

A pioneering leadership study conducted in the late 1930s by Ronald Lippitt and Ralph

K. White under the general direction of Kurt Lewin at the University of Iowa has had a lasting impact. In the initial studies, hobby clubs for ten-year-old boys were formed. Each club was submitted to three different styles of leadership—authoritarian, democratic, and laissez faire. The authoritarian leader was very directive and allowed no participation. This leader tended to give individual attention when praising and criticizing but tried to be friendly or impersonal rather than openly hostile. The democratic leader encouraged group discussion and decision. He tried to be "objective" in his praise or criticism and to be one of the group in spirit. The laissez faire leader gave complete freedom to the group; he essentially provided no leadership.

Under experimental conditions, the three leadership styles were manipulated to show their effects on variables such as satisfaction and frustration-aggression. Controls in the experiment included the following:

1. Characteristics of the boys. All the boys had about the same intelligence and social behaviors.

2. Types of activities performed. Each of the clubs made similar things, such as masks, model airplanes, murals, and soap carvings.

3. The physical setting and equipment. The experiments were conducted in the same

---

†In adapting previously published literature, the editor has added original commentary. Throughout the rest of this book, the editor's contributions are italicized to distinguish them from reprinted material.

rooms and used identical equipment for all the clubs.

4. The physical characteristics and personality of the leader. The leaders assumed a different style as they shifted every six weeks from group to group [1].

These controls were employed so that the experimenters could state with some degree of assurance that the styles of leadership were causing the changes in the dependent variables of satisfaction and frustration-aggression.

RESULTS OF THE STUDIES. Some of the results were clear-cut and others were not. One definite finding was the boys' overwhelming preference for their democratic leader. They said the autocrat "didn't let us do what we wanted to do," or "we just had to do things; he wanted us to get it done in a hurry" [2]. They liked the democratic leader because "he never did try to be the boss, but we always had plenty to do" [3]. The boys also chose the laissez faire leader over the autocratic one in seven out of ten cases. For most of the boys, even confusion and disorder were preferable to strictness and rigidity.

Unfortunately, the effects that styles of leadership had on productivity were not directly examined. The experiments were primarily designed to examine patterns of aggressive behavior. However, an important by-product was the insight that was gained into the productive behavior of a group. For example, the researchers found that the boys subjected to the autocratic leader reacted in one of two ways: either aggressively or apathetically. Through filming and recording detailed observations, Lippitt's original 1937 study found hostility was 30 times as frequent in the autocratic as in the democratic group. Also, aggression ("hostility" and "joking hostility") was eight

times as prevalent. In a second experiment, performed a year later, one of five autocratic groups had the same aggressive reaction. The other four had extremely nonaggressive, "apathetic" patterns of behavior. Both the aggressive and apathetic behaviors were deemed to be reactions to the frustration caused by the autocratic leader. The researchers also pointed out that the apathetic groups exhibited outbursts of aggression when the autocratic leader left the room or when a transition was made to a freer leadership atmosphere. The laissez faire leadership climate actually produced the greatest number of aggressive acts from the group. The democratically led group fell between the one extremely aggressive group and the four apathetic groups under the autocratic leaders.

IMPLICATIONS OF THE STUDIES. Sweeping generalizations on the basis of the Lippitt and White studies are dangerous. From the viewpoint of modern behavioral science research methodology, many of the variables were not controlled. The value of the studies was that they were the first to analyze leadership from the standpoint of scientific methodology and, more important, they showed that different styles of leadership can produce different, complex reactions from the same or similar groups.

Ohio State Leadership Studies

In 1945, the Bureau of Business Research at Ohio State University initiated a series of studies on leadership. An interdisciplinary team of researchers from psychology, sociology, and economics developed and used the Leader Behavior Description Questionnaire (LBDQ) to analyze leadership in numerous types of groups and situations [4]. Studies were made of Air Force commanders and members of bomber crews; officers, noncommissioned personnel, and civilian administrators in the Navy Department; manufacturing foremen; executives of regional cooperatives; college administrators; teachers, principals, and school superintendents; and leaders of various student and civilian groups.

The Ohio State studies started with the premise that no satisfactory definition of leadership existed. They also recognized that previous work had too often assumed that "leadership" was synonymous with "good leadership." The Ohio State group was determined to study leadership, regardless of definition or whether it was effective or ineffective.

In the first step, the LBDQ was administered in various leadership situations. In order to examine the leader's behavior, the answers to the questionnaire were then subjected to factor analysis. The outcome was amazingly consistent. The same two dimensions of leadership behavior continually emerged. The strongest was **consideration** and the next strongest was **initiating structure**. The consideration factor meant that a friendly, trusting, respectful, and warm relationship existed between the leader and the followers. Initiating structure meant that the leader organized and defined the relationship between himself and the members of his crew. "He tends to define the role which he expects each member of the crew to assume, and endeavors to establish well-defined patterns of organization, channels of communication, and ways of getting jobs done" [5]. Combined, consideration and initiating structure accounted for 83.2 percent of the common-factor variance in this study.

The same two factors were found in many follow-up studies encompassing many kinds of leadership positions and contexts. The researchers carefully emphasize that the studies show only **how** leaders carry out their

leadership position. Initiating structure and consideration are very similar to the time-honored military commander's functions of mission and concern with the welfare of the men. In simple terms, the Ohio State factors are task or goal orientation (initiating structure) and recognition of individual needs (consideration). The two dimensions are separate and distinct from one another.

The value of the Ohio State studies is their empirical determination of the functions of leadership. These studies were the first to point out and emphasize the importance of **both** task direction and consideration of individual needs in assessing leadership behavior. This two-dimensional approach lessened the gap between the strict task orientation of the scientific management movement and the human relations emphasis which was popular up to recent times.

Early Michigan Studies on Leadership Styles

At about the same time the Ohio State studies were being conducted, the Office of Naval Research granted a contract to the University of Michigan Survey Research Center. The purpose of the grant was to determine the "principles which contribute both to the productivity of the group and to the satisfaction that the group members derive from their participation" [6]. To accomplish this objective, a study was initiated in 1947 at the home office of the Prudential Insurance Company, Newark, New Jersey.

The Michigan group tried to avoid the methodological difficulties of other pioneering research such as the failure to develop quantitative measures for variables affecting supervisors and workers in the Hawthorne studies. Systematic measurement was made of the perceptions and attitudes of supervisors and workers. These variables were then related to measures of performance. The research design also included a high degree of control over nonpsychological variables that might influence morale and productivity. Thus, certain factors, such as type of work, working conditions, and work methods, were controlled.

Twelve high–low productivity pairs were selected for examination. Each pair represented a high-producing section and a low-producing section, with the other variables, such as type of work, conditions, and methods, being the same in each pair. Nondirective interviews were conducted with the 24 section supervisors and 419 clerical-type workers. Results showed that supervisors of high-producing sections were significantly more likely

1. To receive general, rather than close, supervision from their supervisors

2. To like the amount of authority and responsibility they have in their jobs

3. To spend more time in supervision

4. To give general, rather than close, supervision to their employees

5. To be employee-oriented, rather than production-oriented [7]

The low-producing section supervisors had essentially opposite characteristics and techniques. They were found to be close, production-centered supervisors. Another important, but sometimes overlooked, finding was that employee satisfaction was **not** directly related to productivity.

The general, employee-centered supervisor, described above, has been the standard-bearer for the traditional human relations approach to leadership. The studies have been followed up with hundreds of similar studies in a wide variety of industrial, hospital, governmental, and other organizations. In 1961, Rensis Likert presented the results of the years of research in **New Patterns of Management** [8]. Although there were some variations and refinements, the "new patterns" were essentially the same as those found in the Prudential studies.

THEORIES OF LEADERSHIP

The Lippitt and White, Ohio State, and Michigan studies are three of the historically most important leadership studies for the study of organizational behavior. Unfortunately, they are still heavily depended upon, and leadership research has not surged ahead from this relatively auspicious beginning. Before analyzing the current status of leadership research, it is important to look at the theoretical development that has occurred through the years.

There are several distinct theoretical bases for leadership. At first leaders were felt to be born, not made. This so-called great man theory of leadership implied that some individuals were born with certain traits that allowed them to emerge out of any situation or period of history to become leaders. This evolved into what is now known as the trait theory of leadership. Another approach was to give greater attention to followers. The trait approach is mainly concerned with identifying personality traits of the leader. Because of the dissatisfaction with this approach, and stimulated by research such as the Ohio State studies, emphasis switched from the individual leader to the group being led. In the group approach, leadership is viewed more in terms of the leader's behavior and how such behavior affects and is affected by the group of followers. Finally, besides the leader and the group, the situation began to receive increased attention in leadership theory. The situation was initially called **Zeitgeist** (a German word meaning "spirit of the times"), and the leader is viewed as a product of the times, the situation. The person with the particular qualities or traits that a situation requires will emerge as the leader. Such a view has much historical support for a theoretical base for leadership and serves as the base for today's situational, and now, contingency, theories of leadership. Finally, very recently, some of the expectancy concepts of motivation began to be adapted to leadership. Called the path-goal theory of leadership, this latest approach is a step toward synthesizing motivational and leadership concepts. The following will examine in detail these major theoretical bases of leadership.

Trait Theories of Leadership

The scientific analysis of leadership started off by concentrating on leaders themselves. The vital question that this theoretical approach attempted to answer was, what characteristics or traits make a person a leader? The earliest trait theories, which can be traced back to the ancient Greeks and Romans, concluded that leaders were born, not made. This "great man" theory of leadership said that a person was born either with or without the necessary traits for leadership. Famous figures in history, for example Napoleon, were said to have had the natural leadership abilities to rise out of any situation to be a great leader.

Eventually, the great man theory gave way to a more realistic trait approach to leadership. Under the influence of the behavioristic school of psychological thought, acceptance was given to the fact that leadership traits are not completely inborn but can also be acquired through learning and experience. Attention turned to the search for universal traits possessed by leaders. Numerous physical, mental, and personality traits were researched from about 1930 to 1950. The results of this voluminous research effort were generally very disappointing. Only intelligence seemed to hold up with any degree of consistency.

Almost any adjective can be used to describe a successful leader. Recognizing these semantic limitations and realizing that there is no cause-and-effect relationship between observed traits and successful leadership, Keith Davis summarizes four of the major traits which seem to have an impact on successful organizational leadership [9]:

1. **Intelligence.** Research generally shows that the leader has higher intelligence than the average intelligence of his followers. Interestingly, however, the leader cannot be exceedingly much more intelligent than his followers.

2. **Social maturity and breadth.** Leaders tend to be emotionally stable and mature and to have broad interests and activities. They have an assured, respectful self-concept.

3. **Inner motivation and achievement drives.** Leaders have relatively intense motivational drives of the achievement type. They strive for intrinsic rather than extrinsic rewards.

4. **Human relations attitudes.** A successful leader recognizes the worth and dignity of his followers and is able to empathize with them. In the terminology of the Ohio State leadership studies, he possesses consideration, and in the Michigan studies terminology, he is employee- rather than production-centered.

The preceding represents only one among many possible lists of important organizational leadership traits. Although one can find some research evidence to support the traits on Davis's list and others, to date none are conclusive. Research findings do not begin to agree on which traits are generally found in leaders or even which ones are more important than others. Similar to the trait theories of personality, the trait approach to leadership has provided some descriptive insight but has little analytical or predictive value.

Group Theories of Leadership

The group theories of leadership have their roots in social psychology. Homans' exchange theory, in particular, serves as an important basis for this approach. According to this theory the leader provides more benefits/rewards than burdens/costs for followers. There must be a positive exchange between the leader and followers in order for group goals to be accomplished. Chester Barnard applied such an analysis to managers and subordinates in an organizational setting almost 40 years ago. More recently Hollander and Julian articulate the social exchange view of leadership as follows:

the person in the role of leader who fulfills expectations and achieves group goals provides rewards for others which are reciprocated in the form of status, esteem, and heightened influence. Because leadership embodies a two-way influence relationship, recipients of influence assertions may respond by asserting influence in return. . . . The very sustenance of the relationship depends upon some yielding to influence on both sides. [10]

This quote emphasizes that leadership is an exchange process between the leader and followers and also involves the sociological concept of role expectations. Social psychological research can be used to support the exchange and role concepts applied to leadership. In addition, the original Ohio State studies and follow-up studies through the years, especially the dimension of giving consideration to followers, gives support to the group perspective of leadership. A thorough review of research to date indicates that leaders who take into account and support their followers have a positive impact on attitudes, satisfaction, and performance [11]. However, these findings are tempered by the fact that there are many other variables in the leadership process (for example, the leader's traits and situational variables). All three seem to have an impact on satisfaction and performance and, similarly to the case of motivation, the direction of causality is not clear. The research evidence does not make clear whether the traditionally assumed case that a certain style of leadership (e.g., supportive of the group) leads to or causes satisfaction and performance or the reverse is correct [12].

Situational Theories of Leadership

After both the trait and group approaches proved to fall short of an adequate overall theory of leadership, attention turned to the situational aspects of leadership. Starting in the 1940s, social psychologists began the search for situational variables that impact on leadership roles, skills, and behavior and on followers' performance and satisfaction. Numerous situational variables were identified but no overall situational theory pulled it all together. Then, about a decade ago, Fred Fiedler proposed a situationally based model for leadership effectiveness. A brief review of his research techniques and findings is necessary to fully understand his contingency theory of leadership effectiveness.

ASO AND LPC SCORES. Fiedler developed a unique operational technique to measure leadership style. Measurement is obtained from scores which indicate the Assumed Similarity between Opposites (ASO) and Least Preferred Coworker (LPC). ASO calculates the degree of similarity between leaders' perceptions of their most and least preferred coworkers. LPC calculates the degree to which the leaders favorably perceive their worst coworkers. The two measurements, which can be used interchangeably, relate to leadership style in the following manner:

1. **The human relations or "lenient" style** is associated with the leader who does not

discern a great deal of difference between the most and least preferred coworkers (ASO) **or** who gives a relatively favorable description of the least preferred coworker (LPC).

2. **The task-directed or "hard-nosed" style** is associated with the leader who perceives a great difference between the most and least preferred coworkers (ASO) and gives a very unfavorable description of the least preferred coworker (LPC).

FIEDLER'S FINDINGS. Through the years the performance of both laboratory groups and numerous real groups (basketball teams, fraternity members, surveying teams, bomber crews, infantry squads, open-hearth steel employees, and farm-supply service employees) was correlated with the leadership styles described above. The results were somewhat encouraging, but no simple relationships between leadership style as determined by the leaders' ASO and LPC scores and group performance developed. Eventually Fiedler concluded that more attention would have to be given to situational variables. He became convinced that leadership style in combination with the situation determines group performance.

Fiedler's Contingency Model of Leadership

To test the hypothesis he had formulated from previous research findings, Fiedler developed what he called a contingency model of leadership effectiveness. This model contained the relationship between leadership style and the favorableness of the situation. Situational favorableness was described by Fiedler in terms of three empirically derived dimensions:

1. The **leader-member relationship,** which is the most critical variable in determining the situation's favorableness

2. The degree of **task structure,** which is the second most important input into the favorableness of the situation

3. The leader's **position power** obtained through formal authority, which is the third most critical dimension of the situation [13]

Situations are favorable to the leader if all three of the above dimensions are high. In other words, if the leader is generally accepted by followers (high first dimension), if the task is very structured and everything is "spelled out" (high second dimension), and if a great deal of authority and power is formally attributed to the leader's position (high third dimension), the situation is very favorable. If the opposite exists (if the three dimensions are low), the situation will be very unfavorable for the leader. Fiedler was convinced that the favorableness of the situation in combination with the leadership style determines effectiveness.

Through the manipulation of research findings, Fiedler was able to discover that under very favorable **and** very unfavorable situations, the task-directed or "hard-nosed" type of leader was most effective. However, when the situation was only moderately favorable or unfavorable (the intermediate range of favorableness), the human relations or lenient type of leader was most effective. Exhibit 1-1 summarizes this relationship between leadership style and the favorableness of the situation.

Why is the task-directed type of leader successful in very favorable situations? Fiedler offered the following explanation:

In the very favorable conditions in which the leader has power, informal backing, and a relatively well-structured task, the group is ready to be directed, and the group expects to be told what to do. Consider the captain of an airliner in its final landing approach. We would hardly want him to turn to his crew for a discussion on how to land. [14]

Exhibit 1-1. Fiedler's Model of Leadership

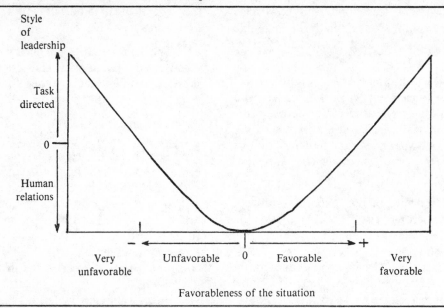

Adapted from *A Theory of Leadership Effectiveness* by Fred E. Fiedler. Copyright © 1967, McGraw-Hill Inc. Used with permission of McGraw-Hill Book Company.

As an example of why the task-oriented leader is successful in a highly unfavorable situation, Fiedler cited

the disliked chairman of a volunteer committee which is asked to plan the office picnic on a beautiful Sunday. If the leader asks too many questions about what the group ought to do or how he should proceed, he is likely to be told that "we ought to go home." [15]

The leader who makes a wrong decision in this highly unfavorable type of situation is probably better off than the leader who makes no decision at all. Exhibit 1-1 shows that the human relations leader is effective in the intermediate range of favorableness. An example of such situations is the typical committee or a unit which is staffed by professionals. In these situations, the leader may not be wholly accepted by the other members of the group, the task may be generally vague and not completely structured, and little authority and power may be granted to the leader. Under such cir-

cumstances, the model predicts that a human relations, lenient type of leader will be most effective.

RESEARCH SUPPORT OF THE CONTINGENCY MODEL. Fiedler's model has stimulated a great deal of research. As is true of most theories in the social-behavioral sciences, the results are mixed and a controversy has been generated. Fiedler himself recognizes that his model must be able to explain and predict if it is to be a valid theory for leadership.

On the basis of 30 studies in a wide variety of teams and organizations, e.g., navy teams, chemical research teams, shop departments, supermarkets, heavy machinery plant departments, engineering groups, hospital wards, public health teams, and others, Fiedler concludes that "the theory is highly predictive and that the relations obtained in the validation studies are almost identical to those obtained in the original studies" [16]. With one exception which

Fiedler explains away, the model correctly predicted the correlations that should exist between LPC scores of the leader (which determines the style) and performance in relation to the identified favorableness of the situation. For example, his studies show that in very unfavorable and very favorable situations, there is a negative correlation between the leader's LPC score and performance (i.e., the task-oriented leader performs best). In a moderately favorable and moderately unfavorable situation, there is a positive correlation between the leader's LPC score and performance (i.e., the human relations-oriented leader is more effective).

CRITICAL ANALYSIS OF THE CONTINGENCY MODEL. Some researchers do not wholly agree with Fiedler's interpretations or conclusions. Most of the justifiable criticism comes from Fiedler's extension of the model to the actual practice of human resource management. Based on the model, Fiedler suggests that management would be better off to engineer positions so that the requirements fit the leader instead of the more traditional way of selecting and developing leaders to fit into existing jobs [17]. Although appealing and with significant potential implications for selection and development of managerial personnel and job design, the evidence is not yet sufficient to justify the implementation of this suggestion to human resource management policy and practice. On the other hand, even the critics would admit that Fiedler has provided one of the major breakthroughs for leadership theory and practice. Further research, especially leading to an understanding of what behavior is actually represented by the LPC response and specifying how the situational moderators will change as the leader asserts influence on subordinates, [18] should put Fiedler's contingency approach on firmer ground so that it can actually guide the future practice of human resource management. In addition,

Fiedler has set an important precedent for the development of contingency models, not just for leadership, but for other management concepts and techniques as well [19].

Path-Goal Leadership Theory

The most recent widely recognized theoretical development for leadership uses the expectancy framework from motivation theory. This is a healthy development because leadership is closely related to motivation on the one hand and power on the other. Any theory which attempts to synthesize the various concepts seems to be a step in the right direction.

Although Georgopoulos and his colleagues at the University of Michigan's Institute for Social Research used path-goal concepts and terminology over two decades ago in analyzing the impact of leadership on performance, the modern development is usually attributed to Martin Evans and Robert House in separate papers [20]. In essence, the path-goal theory attempts to explain the impact that leader behavior has on subordinate motivation, satisfaction, and performance. The theory incorporates four major types or styles of leader behavior [21]. Briefly summarized these are:

1. **Directive leadership.** This style is similar to the Lippitt and White authoritarian leader. Subordinates know exactly what is expected of them and specific directions are given by the leader. There is no participation by subordinates.

2. **Supportive leadership.** Self-explanatory; the leader is friendly and approachable and shows a genuine human concern for subordinates.

3. **Participative leadership.** This leader asks for and uses suggestions from subordinates but still makes the decisions.

4. **Achievement-oriented leadership.** This leader sets challenging goals for subor-

dinates and shows confidence in them to attain these goals and perform well.

The path-goal theory—and here is how it differs in one respect from Fiedler's contingency model—suggests that these various styles can be and actually are used by the same leader in different situations [22]. Two of the situational factors that have been identified so far are the personal characteristics of subordinates and the environmental pressures and demands facing subordinates. With respect to the first situational factor, the theory asserts that,

leader behavior will be acceptable to subordinates to the extent that the subordinates see such behavior as either an immediate source of satisfaction or as instrumental to future satisfaction [23].

And with respect to the second situational factor, the theory states that,

leader behavior will be motivational (e.g., will increase subordinates' effort) to the extent that 1) it makes satisfaction of subordinates' needs contingent on effective performance, and 2) it complements the environment of subordinates by providing the coaching, guidance, support, and rewards which are necessary for effective performance and which may otherwise be lacking in subordinates or in their environment. [24]

Using one of the four styles contingent upon the situational factors as outlined above, the leader attempts to motivate subordinates, in turn leading to their satisfaction and performance. This is specifically done by

1. Recognizing and/or arousing subordinates' needs for outcomes over which the leader has some control

2. Increasing personal payoffs to subordinates for work-goal attainment

3. Making the path to those payoffs easier to travel by coaching and direction

4. Helping subordinates clarify expectancies

5. Reducing frustrating barriers

6. Increasing the opportunities for personal satisfaction contingent on effective performance [25]

In other words, by doing the foregoing the leader attempts to make the path to goals as smooth as possible for subordinates. But to accomplish this path-goal facilitation, the leader must use the appropriate style contingent on the situational variables present.

There has been a recent surge of research on the path-goal theory of leadership. So far, the research has generally been supportive of the theory. For example, a sampling of the research findings, most of which have been made in the last couple of years, indicates that [26]:

1. Studies of seven organizations have found that **leader directiveness** is 1) positively related to satisfactions and expectancies of subordinates engaged in ambiguous tasks, and 2) negatively related to satisfactions and expectancies of subordinates engaged in clear tasks.

2. Studies involving ten different samples of employees found that **supportive leadership** will have its most positive effect on satisfaction for subordinates who work on stressful, frustrating, or dissatisfying tasks.

3. In a major study in an industrial manufacturing organization, it was found that in nonrepetitive ego-involving tasks, employees were more satisfied under **participative leaders** than under nonparticipative leaders.

4. In three separate organizations it was found that for subordinates performing ambiguous-nonrepetitive tasks, the higher the **achievement orientation of the leader,** the more subordinates were confident that their efforts would pay off in effective performance.

Not all studies that have tested path-goal leadership are as clear and supportive as the one just described, but there does seem to be a great deal of early support, and the theory certainly warrants continued research and refinement. Both the Fiedler contingency model and the path-goal approach take into consideration all three important variables in leadership: the leader, the group, and the situation.

Leadership as an Influence System

A truly meaningful and comprehensive approach to leadership would seem to have to incorporate the leader, the group, and the situation. An influence system model can clarify some of the complexities of modern leadership theory. Exhibit 1-2 depicts the heart of leadership to be influence and consists of the systems interaction of the leader, the group, and the situation. Each of the three major subsystems influences, and is influenced by, the other. Thus, the leader influences the group and the group influences the leader; the leader influences the situation and the situation influences the leader; and the group influences the situation and the situation influences the group.

This influence system model seems most accurately to depict what the leadership process is all about. The following paragraphs relate this model and the other theoretical background to the actual styles of leadership and supervision that are used in the practice of human resource management.

LEADERSHIP STYLES

The classic leadership studies previously discussed and the various leadership theories all have direct implications for what style the manager or supervisor uses in human resource management. The terminology "style" is roughly equivalent to the leader's behavior. It is the **way** in which the leader influences followers. The following discussion will first explore the implications for style from the classic studies and the theories, and then it will present the most recent approaches that deal directly with style.

Style Implications from the Classic Studies and the Modern Theories

The Hawthorne studies were interpreted in terms of their implications for supervisory

Exhibit 1-2.   The Influence System Model of Leadership

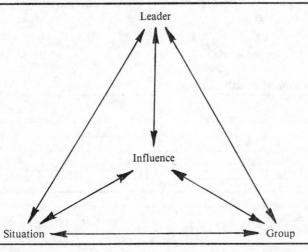

style, and Douglas McGregor's Theory X represents the old, authoritarian style and his Theory Y represents the enlightened, humanistic style of leadership. Also, the studies described in the foregoing were concerned with style. The Lippitt and White study analyzed the impact of autocratic, democratic, and laissez faire styles, and the Prudential studies conducted by the Michigan group found the employee-centered supervisor to be more effective than the production-centered supervisor. The Ohio State studies identified consideration (a supportive type of style) and initiating structure (a directive type of style) as being the major functions of leadership. Both the trait and the group theories have indirect implications for style, and the human relations and task-directed styles play a direct role in Fiedler's contingency theory. The path-goal conceptualization depends heavily upon directive, supportive, participative, and achievement-oriented styles of leadership.

The various styles discussed so far can be incorporated into the continuum shown in Exhibit 1-3. Although this categorization represents only a rough approximation of the various styles for ease of presentation and a brief summary, the styles may be substituted for the boss-centered/subordinate-centered terminology used in Exhibit 1-4. The verbal descriptions and the relation between authority and freedom found in Exhibit 1-4 give an overall rough summary of the characteristics of the various styles of leadership. This depiction can serve as background for a more detailed examination of the specific application of styles to the practice of human resource management.

Managerial Grid Styles

One very popular approach to identifying leadership styles of practicing managers is the use of Robert R. Blake and Jane S. Mouton's managerial grid. Exhibit 1-5 shows that the two dimensions of the grid are concern for people, along the vertical axis, and concern for production, along the horizontal. These two dimensions, of course, are equivalent to the consideration and initiating structure functions identified by the Ohio State studies and the employee-centered and production-centered styles used in the Michigan studies.

The five basic styles identified in the grid represent varying combinations of concern for people and production. The 1, 1 manager has minimum concern for people and production and is sometimes labeled the "impoverished" style. The opposite is the 9, 9 manager. This individual has maximum concern for people and production. Practically all managers feel this is the best style of management, but Blake and Mouton carefully point out that the best style will depend on the situation. The 5, 5 manager is the "middle-of-the-roader," and the other two styles represent the extreme concerns for people (1,9, "country club" manager) and

Exhibit 1-3. Continuum of Leadership Styles

Boss-centered	Subordinate-centered
Theory X	Theory Y
autocratic	democratic
production-centered	employee-centered
close	general
initiating structure	consideration
task-directed	human relations
directive	supportive
directive	participative

Exhibit 1-4. A Continuum of Leadership Behavior

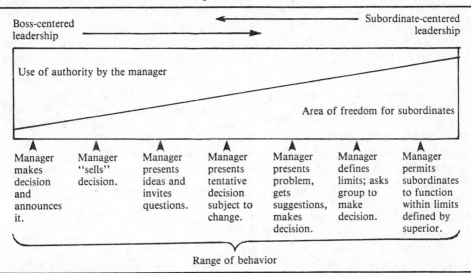

Boss-centered leadership   Subordinate-centered leadership

Use of authority by the manager

Area of freedom for subordinates

| Manager makes decision and announces it. | Manager "sells" decision. | Manager presents ideas and invites questions. | Manager presents tentative decision subject to change. | Manager presents problem, gets suggestions, makes decision. | Manager defines limits; asks group to make decision. | Manager permits subordinates to function within limits defined by superior. |

Range of behavior

From Robert Tannenbaum and Warren H. Schmidt, "How to Choose a Leadership Pattern," *Harvard Business Review,* **March-April 1958, p. 96. Used with permission.**

Exhibit 1-5. The Managerial Grid

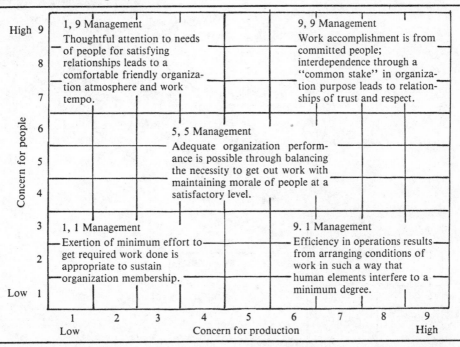

High 9

1, 9 Management
Thoughtful attention to needs of people for satisfying relationships leads to a comfortable friendly organization atmosphere and work tempo.

9, 9 Management
Work accomplishment is from committed people; interdependence through a "common stake" in organization purpose leads to relationships of trust and respect.

5, 5 Management
Adequate organization performance is possible through balancing the necessity to get out work with maintaining morale of people at a satisfactory level.

1, 1 Management
Exertion of minimum effort to get required work done is appropriate to sustain organization membership.

9. 1 Management
Efficiency in operations results from arranging conditions of work in such a way that human elements interfere to a minimum degree.

Low 1

Concern for people

1   2   3   4   5   6   7   8   9
Low   Concern for production   High

Reprinted, by permission of the publisher, from "Managerial Facades" by Robert R. Blake and Jane S. Mouton, *Advanced Management Journal,* **July 1966,** © **1966 by Society for Advancement of Management, p. 31. All rights reserved.**

production (9,1, "task" manager). Where a manager falls on the grid can be determined by a questionnaire developed by Blake and Mouton, and the results can play an important role in organization development.

Reddin's Three-Dimensional Model

Blake and Mouton's grid identifies the style of a manager but does not directly relate it to effectiveness. William J. Reddin, a Canadian professor and consultant, has added the third dimension, effectiveness, to his model. Besides incorporating the effectiveness dimension, he also builds in the situational impact on the appropriate style. Exhibit 1-6 shows the relatively elaborate 3-D leader effectiveness model.

The center grid in Exhibit 1-6 represents the four basic leadership styles. These are basically the same as the styles identified by Blake and Mouton. Importantly, where Reddin goes beyond the Blake and Mouton grid, each of the four styles can be effective or ineffective depending on the situation. The four styles on the upper right are effective (they achieve the output requirements of the manager's job and/or attain the goals of the position) and the four styles on the lower left are ineffective. Very briefly, these eight styles can be summarized as follows [27]:

Effective Styles

1. **Executive.** This style gives a great deal of concern to both task and people. A mana-

Exhibit 1-6.   Reddin's 3-D Model of Leadership Effectiveness

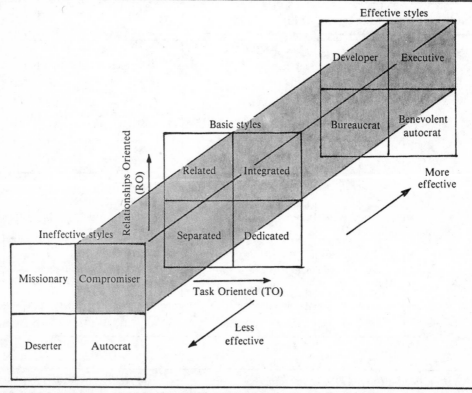

Adapted from *Managerial Effectiveness* by **W.J. Reddin. Copyright © 1970, McGraw-Hill, Inc. Used with permission of McGraw-Hill Book Company.**

ger using this style is a good motivator, sets high standards, recognizes individual differences, and utilizes team management.

2. **Developer.** This style gives maximum concern to people and minimum concern to the task. A manager using this style has implicit trust in people and is mainly concerned with developing them as individuals.

3. **Benevolent Autocrat.** This style gives maximum concern to the task and minimum concern to people. A manager using this style knows exactly what he or she wants and how to get it without causing resentment.

4. **Bureaucrat.** This style gives minimum concern to both task and people. A manager using this style is mainly interested in the rules and wants to maintain and control the situation by their use but is seen as conscientious.

Ineffective Styles

1. **Compromiser.** This style gives a great deal of concern to both task and people in a situation that requires only emphasis on one or neither. This style of manager is a poor decision maker; the pressures affect him or her too much.

2. **Missionary.** This style gives maximum concern to people and minimum concern to the task where such behavior is inappropriate. This manager is typically the "do gooder" who values harmony as an end in itself.

3. **Autocrat.** This style gives maximum concern to the task and minimum concern to the people where such behavior is inappropriate. This manager has no confidence in others, is unpleasant, and is interested only in the immediate job.

4. **Deserter.** This style gives minimum concern to task and people in a situation where such behavior is inappropriate. This manager is uninvolved and passive.

Likert's Four Systems of Management

Both the Blake and Mouton and the Reddin 3-D approaches are highly descriptive and at this time lack empirically validated research back-up. In contrast, on the basis of the many years of research by the Michigan group, Rensis Likert proposes four basic systems or styles of organizational leadership. Exhibit 1-7 summarizes these four styles.

The manager who operates under a system 1 approach is very authoritarian and actually tries to exploit subordinates. The system 2 manager is also authoritarian but in a paternalistic manner. This benevolent autocrat keeps strict control and never delegates to subordinates, but he or she "pats them on the head" and "does it for their best interests." The system 3 manager uses a consultative style. This manager asks for and receives participative input from subordinates but maintains the right to make the final decision. The system 4 manager uses a democratic style. This manager gives some direction to subordinates but provides for total participation and decision by consensus and majority.

To give empirical research back-up to determine which style is most effective, Likert and his colleagues asked thousands of managers to describe, on an expanded version of the format shown in Exhibit 1-7, the highest- and lowest-producing departments with which they have had experience. Quite consistently, the high-producing units are described according to systems 3 and 4, and the low-producing units fall under systems 1 and 2. This response occurs irrespective of the manager's field of experience or whether the manager is in a line or staff position [28].

THE IMPACT OF INTERVENING VARIABLES AND TIME. An important refinement of Likert's work is the recognition of three broad classes of variables that affect the relationship between leadership and per-

Exhibit 1-7.   Likert's Systems of Management Leadership

Leadership Variable	System 1 (Exploitive Autocratic)	System 2 (Benevolent Autocratic)	System 3 (Participative)	System 4 (Democratic)
Confidence and trust in subordinates	Has no confidence and trust in subordinates	Has condescending confidence and trust, such as master has to servant	Substantial but not complete confidence and trust; still wishes to keep control of decisions	Complete confidence and trust in all matters
Subordinates' feeling of freedom	Subordinates do not feel at all free to discuss things about the job with their superior	Subordinates do not feel very free to discuss things about the job with their superior	Subordinates feel rather free to discuss things about the job with their superior	Subordinates feel completely free to discuss things about the job with their superior
Superiors seeking involvement with subordinates	Seldom gets ideas and opinions of subordinates in solving job problems	Sometimes gets ideas and opinions of subordinates in solving job problems	Usually gets ideas and opinions and usually tries to make constructive use of them	Always asks subordinates for ideas and opinions and always tries to make constructive use of them

Adapted from *The Human Organization* by Rensis Likert. Copyright © 1967, McGraw-Hill, Inc. Used with permission of McGraw-Hill Book Company.

formance in a complex organization [29]. Briefly summarized, these are:

1. **Causal variables.** These are the independent variables that determine the course of developments and results of an organization. They include only those variables that are under control of management; e.g., economic conditions are **not** causal variables in this sense. Examples would include organization structure and management's policies and decisions and their leadership styles, skills, and behavior.

2. **Intervening variables.** These reflect the internal climate of the organization. Performance goals, loyalties, attitudes, perceptions, and motivations are some important

intervening variables. They affect interpersonal relations, communication, and decision-making in the organization.

3. **End-result variables.** These are the dependent variables, the outcomes of the organization. Examples would be productivity, service, costs, quality, and earnings.

Importantly, Likert points out that there is not a direct cause-and-effect relationship between, for example, leadership style (a causal variable) and earnings (an end-result variable). The intervening variables must also be taken into consideration. For example, moving to a system 1 style of management may lead to an improvement in profits but a deterioration of the intervening variables (i.e., attitudes, loyalty, and motivation decline). In time, these intervening variables may lead to a decrease in profits. Thus, although on the surface it appeared that system 1 was causing profits, because of the impact on the intervening variables, in the long run system 1 may lead to a decrease in profits. The same can be said for the application of a system 4 style. In the short run, profits may dip; but because of the impact on intervening variables, there will be an increase in profit over time. Obviously, the time lag between intervention and the impact on end-result variables becomes extremely important to Likert's scheme. Based upon some research evidence, Likert concludes that, "Changes in the causal variables toward System 4 apparently require an appreciable period of time before the impact of the change is fully manifest in corresponding improvement in end-result variables" [30].

AN EXAMPLE OF TIME LAG. Likert's "time-lag" helps explain the following relatively common sequence of events. A system 1 manager takes over an operation and immediately gets good performance results. In the meantime, however, the in-

tervening variables are declining. Because the system 1 manager is getting results, he is promoted. A system 4 manager now takes over the operation. Because of the time lag, the intervening variables, which were affected by the system 1 manager, now start to impact on performance. Under the system 4 manager, performance starts to decline but the intervening variables start to improve. However, top management sees that when the system 4 manager took over, performance started to decline. The system 4 manager is replaced by a system 1 manager to "tighten up" the operation. The intervening variables affected by the system 4 manager now start to affect performance and the cycle repeats. Exhibit 1-8 graphically depicts this situation. In other words, the cause-and-effect relationships that appear on the surface may be very misleading because of the time-lag impact of the intervening variables. As in the example, top-management evaluations often credit the wrong manager (the system 1 manager in this case) for improving performance and unjustly blame the wrong manager (the system 4 manager in the example) for poor performance. Some organizations are caught up in this never-ending cycle of rewarding and

Exhibit 1-8. (Hypothetical Example Depicting Likert's Time-Lag Impact of Intervening Variables on Performance)

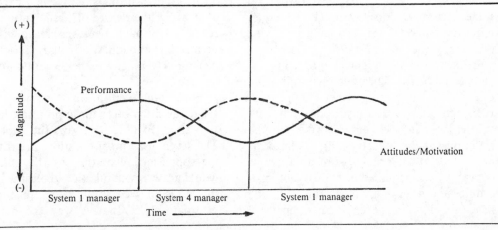

punishing the wrong managers because of the time-lag effect of intervening variables.

ANALYSIS OF LIKERT'S APPROACH. Likert and his colleagues are still actively involved in further development, research, and application of the system 4 style of management. For example, some predictive models are being developed to forecast what impact current causal and intervening variables will have on future outcome variables such as profit.

One of the major criticisms of Likert's work is the overdependence on survey questionnaire measures for gathering data to develop the theory and application of system 4 management. Sole dependence on Likert scale (continuums of dimensions as shown in Exhibit 1-7) questionnaire responses is not enough. Multiple measures of behaviorally oriented variables in organizations are needed. Use of archival information (existing records kept by every organization for other use, e.g., government reports, personnel records, and performance data) and data gathered through observation are needed. Although ethical standards must always be maintained, subject awareness must be minimized to increase the reliability and validity of data that are gathered for research purposes. Both questionnaires and interviews have a great deal of subject awareness or intrusiveness. Archives and some naturalistic observational techniques minimize subject awareness and are called **unobtrusive measures** [31].

Besides the measurement problems inherent in Likert's scheme is the implication of the universality of the system 4 approach. Although Likert carefully points out that "differences in the kind of work, in the traditions of the industry, and in the skills and values of the employees of a particular company will require quite different procedures and ways to apply appropriately the basic principles of system 4 management,"

[32] he still implies that system 4 will **always** be more effective than system 1. The situational/contingency leadership theories and research findings would, of course, counter this generalization.

The Vroom-Yetton Normative Model

The Blake and Mouton, Reddin, and Likert approaches to leadership are all directly or by implication prescriptive. In addition, to varying degrees they try to take into consideration the situation (Blake and Mouton and Likert in passing and Reddin as a vital part of his approach). But none of these approaches spell out exactly **how** a manager should act or what decision should be made in a given situation. Vroom and Yetton attempt to provide a specific, normative (how decisions "ought" to be made in given situations) model that a leader could actually use in making effective decisions [33].

The Vroom-Yetton model was first developed several years ago and has since been modified. The latest model contains five leadership styles, seven situation dimensions, 14 problem types, and seven decision rules. The leadership styles consist of variations of autocratic, consultative, and group styles and the situational dimensions are of two general types: 1) the way in which problems affect the quality and acceptance of a decision, and 2) the way in which the problems affect the degree of participation. The seven situational dimensions are stated in the form of yes-no questions and the answers can quickly diagnose the situation for the leader.

Vroom and Yetton use a decision tree to relate the situation to the appropriate leadership style. Exhibit 1-9 shows the approach. The seven situational questions are listed at the top. Starting at the left, the manager would answer each question above the box in the decision tree until it led to the appropriate style. In this way the manager

Exhibit 1-9. Vroom-Yetton Normative Leadership Model

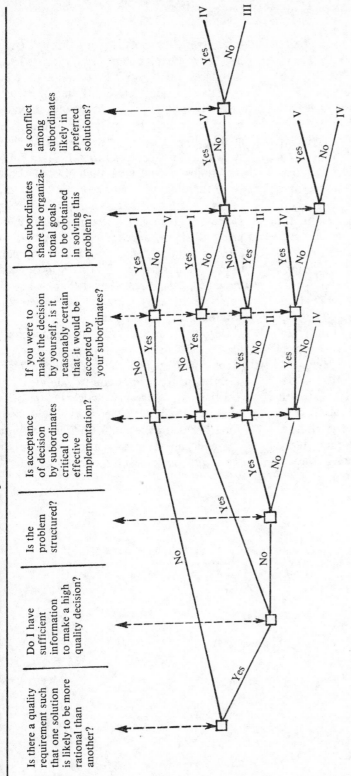

| Is there a quality requirement such that one solution is likely to be more rational than another? | Do I have sufficient information to make a high quality decision? | Is the problem structured? | Is acceptance of decision by subordinates critical to effective implementation? | If you were to make the decision by yourself, is it reasonably certain that it would be accepted by your subordinates? | Do subordinates share the organizational goals to be obtained in solving this problem? | Is conflict among subordinates likely in preferred solutions? |

I. You solve the problem or make the decision yourself, using information available to you at that time. **II.** You obtain the necessary information from your subordinate(s), then decide on the solution to the problem yourself. You may or may not tell your subordinates what the problem is in getting the information from them. The role played by your subordinates in making the decision is clearly one of providing the necessary information to you, rather than generating or evaluating alternative solutions. **III.** You share the problem with relevant subordinates individually, getting their ideas and suggestions without bringing them together as a group. Then **you** make the decision that may or may not reflect your subordinates' influence. **IV.** You share the problem with your subordinates as a group, collectively obtaining their ideas and suggestions. Then **you** make the decision that may or may not reflect your subordinates' influence. **V.** You share a problem with your subordinates as a group. Together you generate and evaluate alternatives and attempt to reach agreement (consensus) on a solution. Your role is much like that of a chairperson. You do not try to influence the group to adopt "your" solution and you are willing to accept and implement any solution that has the support of the entire group.

Adapted and reprinted, by permission of the publisher, from "A New Look at Managerial Decision Making," Victor H. Vroom, *Organizational Dynamics*, **Volume 1, Number 4,** © **1973 by AMACOM, a division of American Management Associations, pp. 67, 70. All rights reserved.**

could determine the appropriate style based on the given confronting situation. Vroom and Yetton also point out that the 14 problem types (the combinations of the seven situational variables listed as 1 through 14 in the decision tree) could actually have more than one acceptable leadership style. In order to be acceptable, the style must meet the criteria of seven decision rules that protect quality and acceptance. If more than one style remains after the test of both quality and acceptance (and many do), the third most important aspect of a decision—the amount of time—is used to determine the single style that "ought" to be used in the given situation. The styles shown at the ends of the various branches on the decision tree reflect the single best style that should be used in light of the way the situation was diagnosed by answers to the questions at the top.

The Vroom-Yetton model is a fitting conclusion to the discussion of leadership in this chapter. The progression has been from theory to styles to specific prescription. Vroom has used a self-report and standardized problem method of testing his model on over 1000 managers going through training and development programs. These managers were asked to recall a problem they had encountered and to indicate which of the five styles they used to solve it. In the other approach the managers were given standardized problem cases and asked which style could best be used to solve it. One of the major conclusions that Vroom draws from these data is that there are bigger differences **within** managers than there are **between** managers [34]. The managers report using all styles, depending on the situation. Such a finding has implications for contingency management. If true, it means that managers can adapt; they are not so set in one style that they cannot change when confronted with another situation.

Despite the surface logic of the model and the fact that it does give precise answers to practicing managers, the research conducted so far is far from sufficient to validate it and justify its use in actual practice. On the other hand, it certainly is a step in the right direction of bridging the gap from theory to practice and can serve as a prototype for the actual practice of contingency management.

FOUR THEORIES OF LEADERSHIP

By Carol Grangaard Heimann

Reprinted with permission from *The Journal of Nursing Administration*, Volume VI, Number 5, June 1976, pp. 18–24.

[A leader is] the person who helps the group attain objectives by influencing the members of the group to organize their efforts toward the achievement of their goal or goals [35].

Leadership is the ability to influence the behavior of others in order to accomplish the task of a group or to achieve the goals of a group while, at the same time, maintaining the integrity and morale of the group [36].

[A leader is the] individual in the group given the task of directing and coordinating task-relevant group activities or who, in the absence of a designated leader, carries the primary responsibility for performing these functions in the group [37].

Leadership is, by definition, an interpersonal relationship in which power and influence are unevenly distributed so that one person is able to direct and control the actions and behavior of others to a greater extent than they direct and control his [38].

[A] leader is one who represents a dynamic force within a group; and that force is a principal factor in directing the group toward the purposes or goals of the participants [39].

Leadership can be defined as a personal relationship in which one individual directs, coordinates and supervises others in the performance of a common task [40].

To lead . . . means to influence people deliberately and successfully [41].

Effective leadership behavior is "fusing" the individual and the organization in such a way that both simultaneously obtain **optimum** self-actualization [42].

Leadership is the activity of influencing people to cooperate toward some goal which they come to find desirable [43].

To generalize from this handful of the available definitions, the leader is seen as a specific person in a group who influences and directs the other members of the group toward achievement of the tasks or goals of the group. **Leadership is a relationship between the leader and the group members in which the leader directs, controls, and supervises members to achieve the goals of the group and this achievement is satisfying to both leader and group.**

UNIVERSAL THEORIES OF LEADERSHIP

Having defined a leader and leadership, we can now examine three theories of leadership widely used today. Then we will look at a fourth theory, which is a synthesis of the first three. The three theories are style, trait, and situation.

Style Theory of Leadership

By **style** is meant the manner in which leadership is carried out. Perhaps the best known are **autocratic, democratic,** and **laissez faire.** Less well known but worth discussing briefly are the **paternalistic** and **participative** styles.

The autocratic style is also known as authoritarian. The autocratic leader is task-oriented and seeks obedience from the group so that goals can be accomplished. He decides on the goals for the group to accomplish and on the methods and stages of goal attainment, deciding which comes first, second, and last. As the leader, he identifies when the group has reached their goal. The autocrat determines policy for the group. He leads in terms of his own wishes and desires without consulting group members. He is the initiator.

As a result of his actions, the autocrat can create increased hostility and rivalry within his group, identification with the leader role rather than with the group, anxiety about the future, aggression toward others, the need for scapegoats within the group, and rigid behavior by group members [44]. Communication patterns in the group are generally member to leader rather than member to member. There is less group cohesion, decreased individual morale, and lower group productivity.

Usually, the autocratic leader believes himself to be a leader and rarely acknowledges his own doubts or mistakes. He may be ruthless and without consideration for the feelings of group members. The two most positive statements to be made about the autocratic style of leadership is that it is used fairly widely and it is generally effective in crisis situations.

Paternalistic leadership is closely related to autocratic. The group is dependent on the leader, who makes all decisions because he is responsible for group action and wants to prevent mistakes, thus protecting himself and the group. The paternal leader considers the welfare of his group more than the autocrat does. This consideration is the main distinction between autocratic and paternalistic styles of leadership.

At the opposite end of the control continuum is democratic leadership. In this style the group reserves for itself the final authority to make decisions. These decisions arise from the needs of the group and are freely discussed by the members. The group has two rights: self-direction and self-actualization. With the help of the leader, the group sets policies, establishes goals, and decides on steps toward goal achievement. Group members are free to initiate tasks and interactions independently of the leader. The group, not the leader, decides when goals have been accomplished.

Successful functioning of democratic leadership depends on the personal contacts among group members. The leader must have patience to let the group function at its own pace, and the group members must be educated for the process to work. They should have a basic understanding of group dynamics as well as knowledge of the work which they are performing to decide which goals are realistic and of high priority.

Democratic leaders create increased feelings of cohesiveness among group members, an increase in group productivity, greater job satisfaction and morale, a broader time perspective, more flexible behavior of members, fewer feelings of hostility, frustration, and submission, a decrease in the number of complaints, and less of a need for scapegoats [45]. The work which is done may well be more original, since it is the product of several minds rather than just one. The group members tend to be spontaneous, friendly, and liable to make suggestions to each other and the leader. The main problem with democratic leadership occurs when the group members cannot function in the manner described.

Participative leadership is similar to democratic leadership except that the leader ultimately makes decisions for the group. The members are allowed and encouraged to make suggestions, discuss issues, and participate in problem-solving, but the leader decides.

self-esteem ?
in members

Laissez faire or free-rein leadership is in between autocratic and democratic in terms of control by the leader. **Laissez faire style is individual-centered,** while **autocratic style is leader-centered** and **democratic style is group-centered.** The laissez faire leader provides materials and information to the group while exercising minimal control. He serves basically as an information booth, answering questions only when asked. He makes no attempt to evaluate the work performed, either by praise or criticism. The group has freedom of action.

The laissez faire style creates tension and anxiety when subordinates are frustrated by the lack of leadership. The result can be chaos, confusion, and uncertainty [46]. The group is disorganized and its members feel dissatisfied with group performance. Less work is done, and that work is usually of poorer quality than under another style of leadership.

In democratic leadership, the leader is an active member of the group; in laissez faire leadership, the leader is an inactive resource person.

All these styles can be used, depending on the conditions present and the people being led. These styles of leadership are not mutually exclusive in the sense that every leader masters only one. Uris writes that the skillful leader is one who knows which style to use at which time [47].

Trait Theory of Leadership

In the trait theory of leadership the leader is considered to have superior qualities which differentiate him from his followers.

Bernard listed ten categories of traits which a good leader must have and included a reason for each category [48]. In direct contact, a leader must have a striking physical personality. An attractive leader should be large and strong in body and character, since from childhood we are conditioned to respect size and strength. He should have the power of ready speech, especially in repartee, so that he can extricate himself from embarrassing situations. In indirect contact, the leader must have a good voice for speeches and use the media to his advantage.

Because emotional appeals are stronger than rational ones, a leader should be sympathetic, understanding, and friendly. Kindness and helpfulness are more important than competence, as evidenced by the successful leadership of political bosses. A leader should practice justice and humanitarianism on a personal rather than abstract level, since people relate on the more concrete personal level.

When a leader shows honesty and good faith, he is devoted to the cause of the group. He must be careful not to seem better than the group in the sense of giving his allegiance to a higher cause. And, if the group must choose, they would prefer the leader to be identified with the cause rather than to be honest. The successful leader possesses insight both into general human nature and into the nature of the particular people he is leading. Along with insight go courage and persistence to face opposition. The leader must use independent judgment so that he is convinced of his rightness even when opposed. This persistence must be tempered with realism so that he knows when to give in.

A good leader has a balance of good natural ability, originality, good intellectual training, soundness of judgment, mental flexibility, and forethought. In addition to these, he should also possess a cheerful and even temper, poise, experience, self-confidence, and organizing and executive ability. The leader should have moral vision, idealism, the desire to improve others, and unselfishness. Finally, the leader must possess the powers of inhibition and self-discipline so that he is neither headstrong nor impulsive.

Bernard concludes his discussion by acknowledging that few leaders possess all these traits [49].

Tead also compiled a list of traits [50]. He felt that they could be cultivated with varying degrees of success. He did recognize that the list was arbitrary, but hoped that it would present a comprehensive model of the qualifications needed by a leader.

He states that the first requisite for a leader is more than the usual amount of physical and nervous energy. The leader's energy translates itself to his followers and also enables him to persevere when facing opposition. Second is a sense of purpose and direction. This includes knowing both his personal objectives and those of the group. Next comes a feeling of enthusiasm for the purpose of the group, which must be real and results from a feeling of being commanded by a power and strength which the leader in turn commands.

The fourth trait is one of friendliness, affection, and solicitude for the followers, shown by what the leader does and how he does it. Fifth on Tead's list is integrity. Followers must trust the leader and he must conform to the standards and morals of his followers.

Technical mastery is the next quality needed. This involves an ability to formulate, transmit, interpret, and supervise the working out of policies with the people being led. The leader needs to know how long a task should take and how to judge whether a task has been done well or poorly. The leader who displays decisiveness is one who makes decisions and acts so that the job will get done. He uses the scientific method of thinking to make his decisions and is willing to take responsibility for his acts and decisions.

The eighth quality needed is intelligence. Tead sees this as an ability to appraise the situation readily, to see the significance of the situation, and to obtain cues from the situation for appropriate action. An intelligent leader will be versatile, have more ideas, and display a sense of humor.

As a teacher, the leader must set goals, pose problems, and guide the activities of his followers. He is a teacher, not a boss, and must allow the followers to participate in the learning. The last quality needed is faith in people and in the meaning of life. Tead says this is an active effort to bring good to pass and a belief that the effort is worth making [51].

Situation Theory of Leadership

Situation theory holds that the leader is the "individual who happens to be in the position to institute change when history is ready for change" [52]. In other words, the leader is in the right group at the right time and place. **Leadership is a function of the situation, the culture, context, and customs of the group.** Brown says that research demonstrates the need for a situation to be correct if leadership is to be effective [53]. This is verified by the fact that there are many people in history whose ideas were applied only after they died. They tried to lead in an incorrect historical situation. For example, Semmelweiss believed that doctors should wash their hands between dissections and deliveries to decrease the incidence of puerperal fever [54]. In his lifetime, he was scorned and ridiculed by the medical profession for his idea of asepsis. Now he is recognized as a pioneer in this area.

In situation theory, group performance is related to the degree to which the situation provides the leader with an opportunity to exert influence on the group.

Gibb sees situations as having four elements: 1) the structure of the interpersonal relationships within the group, 2) characteristics of the group, 3) the characteristics of the total culture in which the group exists and from which members are drawn, and 4) the physical conditions and task confronting the group. He says a group member becomes the group leader only for the length of time during which he can demonstrate that he is contributing more toward achievement of the group goal than any other group member [55].

Brown blends situational and field theory. Leadership and the leader are both part of a social field. The leader is not separated from the group but is regarded as occupying a position of high potential within the group. His actions are the result of changes in the field structure and are limited by it. The leader is not seen as a catalyst or initiator of change. Rather, **the lines of force in the field center in the leader's position.** When the field changes, his position also changes. This then results in a change of all forces in the field in the direction in which the leader has changed.

Brown believes that the successful leader operates within five laws, which are criteria against which to measure his success. He says the field structure is fluid and this precludes a response to a leader on the basis of his style or traits. The style and traits change less than the field, which thus serves as the logical measure of leadership success [56].

The five field-dynamic laws of leadership [57]:

1. The successful leader must have membership in the group he is attempting to lead. He must have the same attitudes and reaction tendencies as other members.

2. The leader must represent a region of high potential in the social field. He must be of the group in ideals and aims yet also be viewed by the group as being superior. He cannot be viewed as outside of the group but must be viewed as being somewhat above the group or he will be rejected. This position of the leader—of the group and above the group—results in ambivalent feelings of the group toward the leader. The group usually will combine feelings of love and respect for being one of them with fear and hate for being above them.

3. The leader must realize what is the existing field structure and fall in with it to succeed.

4. The successful leader realizes what the long-term trends in field structure are and changes with them. This condition is necessary if the leader is going to succeed at more than the immediate situation.

5. The leader must realize that his leadership increases in potency at the cost of a decrease in freedom. The leader controls the field and the field controls the leader. A leader has more potential in a highly structured field, yet this same field limits his freedom because of the high structure.

A NEW THEORY OF LEADERSHIP—INTERACTION

Acting on the assumption that leadership is a phenomenon which can be explained, there is a newer theory which provides a logical and adequate explanation. This is the interaction theory, which states that a person becomes a leader not only because of personality (this includes style and trait) but also because of the situation. In other words, the explanatory variables are the personality, the situation, **and** the interaction between them.

Interaction theory includes consideration of the followers. As Stogdill says, "the pattern of personal characteristics of the leader must bear some relevant relationship to the characteristics, activities, and goals of the followers" [58]. There is a two-way flow of effects; leader behavior conditions the response of the followers, and follower behavior conditions the response of the leader.

Thus, leadership involves a working relationship between the group members and the leader, who acquires leadership status through active participation and demonstration of his capabilities for completing, or helping the group to complete, cooperative tasks.

Interaction accommodates consideration of the changing nature of these two variables. The situation changes more often and more rapidly than does the leader's personality. By means of interaction group members "work through" many changes, such as a change in goals, a change in group membership, a change in patterns of interactions, or a change in the task facing the group, as when a new coronary care unit is opened or primary nursing is instituted as the means of delivering care where previously team nursing was used. The working conditions of the group may change, as by a move into a new building or a change in the staffing pattern.

The interaction theory seems to be a logical way of considering the problem of leadership—what it is and who is a leader. As a synthesis of the theories of style, trait, and situation, it is comprehensive and permits generalization to any area in which leadership is involved. It can be a useful tool not only for those who function as leaders but also for those who aspire to be leaders. It directs us to look at our own personalities as well as to assess the situations in which we find ourselves. These two appraisals must be done continuously and the results integrated with our knowledge of the various leadership tactics we can adopt.

A PROFILE OF LEADERSHIP AND MOTIVATION WITHIN A CLOSED HOSPITAL CLIMATE

By Steven H. Appelbaum

Reprinted with permission from *Health Care Management Review*, Winter 1978. Published by Aspen Systems Corporation, Germantown, Maryland.

Individual growth among hospital employees can only be recognized and realized when trainees begin to make meaningful, rational decisions in complex hospital situations; a resistive administrative climate stifles individual development. Yet, protectiveness is often exhibited in hospitals, making learning and working less satisfying, less meaningful, and resulting in aborted goals.

To determine the supervisors' readiness for a management development program, a study of leadership styles and motivations was conducted to examine the current climate within a 300-bed northeastern hospital.

TOOLS FOR SOLVING PROBLEMS

The program was intended to provide the participants with tools to be used within their domains of responsibility so they would be able to understand their administrative role, need to communicate, leadership, decision making, problem solving, motivation and management of change-conflict. The tools also provided better understanding of women's roles in the management process and the management-by-objectives system.

An added objective of the program was to develop team-building skills most essential in an interdependent structure and dynamic climate representative of a hospital.

It was most important to determine whether the supervisory personnel felt they were capable of applying new theories and practices in solving real problems within the hospital. This capability was dependent upon these individuals perceiving the administrative climate in the hospital as being open, supportive, trusting, and rewarding. If the trainees perceived the climate to be closed, then developmental failure would intensify fear and anxiety.

SUPERVISORY STYLES

The styles of 90 supervisors were examined in order to gain some insight into the managerial philosophies of hospital supervisors. A McGregor X-Y questionnaire was administered to the 90 trainees in order to determine how they perceived themselves in relation to the job of managing human resources [59].

McGregor's concern for developing the professional manager implied that any growth in this direction must begin with an examination of the perceptions of the manager concerning the nature of individuals. The starting point is a set of fundamental beliefs or assumptions about what people are like. To illustrate two differing views, two theoretical constructs on human nature were developed in relation to work: Theory X and Theory Y—names chosen arbitrarily as neutral designations.

Theory X

Theory X is identified as management's conventional conception of harnessing human energy to organizational requirements. It assumes:

1. Average humans have an inherent dislike of work, and will avoid it if they can.

2. Because of their dislike of work, average humans must be coerced, controlled, directed or threatened with punishment to get them to put forth adequate effort toward the achievement of organizational objectives.

3. Average humans prefer to be directed, wish to avoid responsibility, have relatively little ambition and want security above all.

These assumptions about human nature form, in very large measure, the rationale for management's approach to developing organizational structures, policies and practices.

Hard vs. Soft Management

Hard, or strong, management is characterized by its use of coercion and threat of punishment to obtain the behavior it desires from its people. Tight controls and close supervision are seen as natural accompaniments.

Soft, or weak, management is exemplified in management's conception of its job as one of satisfying people's demands, being ex-

tremely permissive and generally trying to keep harmony in the organization.

The hard approach is seen as producing restricted production output, antagonism ("force breeds counterforce"), militant unionism, and subtle but effective undermining of management's objectives.

Soft management is envisioned as resulting in management's abdication of its responsibilities, producing harmonious but ineffective employees—an indolent work force that continually expects more but gives less and less.

Both hard and soft management are irrelevant because they either ignore or misinterpret the findings of behavioral research, particularly in the area of human motivation. Direction and control, whether accomplished through the hard or soft approach, are held to be inadequate for the motivation of people whose needs are primarily social and egoistic.

Theory X has been the traditionally accepted mode of thinking about productivity and motivation, because management has confused **consequences** with cause and effect. Theory X neither explains human nature nor describes it; instead, Theory X assumptions merely demonstrate what happens to people and production as a consequence of management's adoption of this philosphy.

Theory Y

Theory Y is the embodiment of a set of assumptions about people that are quite different from those of traditional management philosophy. These assumptions include the following:

1. The expenditure of physical and mental effort in work is as natural as play or rest.

2. External control and the threat of punishment are not the only means of getting people to work toward the organiza-

tion's objectives. People will exercise self-direction and self-control toward achieving objectives to which they are committed.

3. Commitment to objectives is a function of the rewards associated with their achievement (esteem and self-actualization, for example).

4. Average people learn, under proper conditions, not only to accept but to seek responsibility.

5. Most people are capable of a relatively high degree of imagination, ingenuity, and creativity in solving organizational problems.

6. Under the conditions of contemporary industrial life, the average person's intellectual potentialities are utilized only partially.

Clearly, the assumptions in Theory Y are optimistic and humanistic. They also reflect an unlimited potential for personal and organizational growth. While Theory X represents a static and somewhat pessimistic view of human nature, Theory Y emerges as dynamic and amenable to the changing nature of organizations and individuals.

Management Must Take Responsibility

If people behave toward their work in the manner that Theory X assumes, the organization is at fault, not the employees, because people are not basically lazy, indifferent, uncooperative, or uncreative. The "negative" behavior of Theory X is one fundamentally **created** by management through its excessive degree of control. If people behave in such a way as to validate the assumptions under Theory X, management uses the behavior (in a circular reasoning process) to rationalize ineffective performance. Under Theory Y, management must be ingenious enough to tap the hidden potential of its work force through the

development of the inherent need of people to be self-motivated and self-controlled.

Control—External vs. Internal

Central to any discussion of the two theories is the matter of control. Under Theory X, control is **externally** imposed upon the individual by management's supervision and atmosphere of constraint. Under Theory Y, the emphasis is on self-control or **internally** controlled employees. Theory Y implies that, within a climate of trust and respect, employees are capable of putting forth willing effort and are capable of controlling their work habits. This point, carried a step further, leads to the principle of **integration**, or the theory that the individuals' needs (for meaningful work, personal freedom, esteem, and creative expression, implicit under Theory Y) can best be met by directing their energies toward the organization's goals. The achievement of this meshing assumes that the organization can be significantly more effective if it recognizes human needs and makes adjustments to meet these needs.

Study Results

Ninety supervisory personnel participated in the X-Y study. On a total scale of from 1X to 20X, 60, or 67 percent, had a range of scores which fell between 2X and 13X with the mean score at 7X. The "X" scale corresponds to the Theory X philosophy just described. (See Exhibit 1-10.)

On a scale of from 1Y to 20Y, 30, or 33 percent, of the supervisors fell between 1Y and 10Y with the mean score at 3Y. The average score recorded on the McGregor X-Y scale was a 5X. This indicates that supervisors are not truly sensitized and committed to the philosophy of Theory Y, but endorse a more rigid posture in actualizing goals within the institution.

Exhibit 1-10.   X-Y Scale

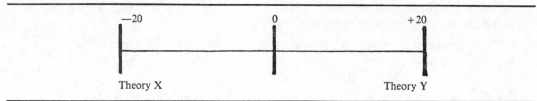

LEADERSHIP BEHAVIOR

Leadership behavior should occupy an equal position between two major variables: consideration and structure.

Structure

While the main focal point of the study was consideration, it was essential to describe structure as measured by the Ohio State Leadership Scale developed by Stogdill and designed to measure the behavior patterns of supervisory and management personnel on both leadership dimensions [60].

Structure reflects the extent to which supervisors exhibit the behavior of leaders in organizing and defining the relationships between themselves and the group, defining interactions among group members, establishing ways of getting the job done, scheduling and criticizing. A high score on the Ohio State Leadership Scale in this dimension describes supervisors who play very active roles in directing group activities through planning, supplying data, trying out new ideas and others. A low score characterizes managers who are likely to be inactive in giving direction in these ways.

Consideration

Consideration reflects the extent to which managers exhibit behavior indicative of mutual trust, respect, friendship, and a positive human relationship toward group or departmental members. A high score on this dimension indicates a climate of good rapport and two-way communication, while a low score indicates an impersonal posture taken by a manager. Both structure and consideration are behaviors which are relatively independent but not necessarily incompatible.

Consideration is not actually a leadership trait, but describes the behavior of leaders in certain situations in an empirical question that is still virtually unanswered. The general norms developed by the Ohio State Leadership Study suggested an average score on consideration to be 44 and an average score for structure to be 40. The higher score for consideration has a relation to the McGregor scale in which a ''Y'' emphasis is considered to be more effective and satisfying than the traditional ''X'' philosophy.

The average score recorded at the hospital for consideration was 45 (one unit more than the norm), but the average score for initiating structure was 46—one unit more than the consideration score but six units higher than the norms developed at Ohio State. This score corroborates the average ''X'' on the McGregor scale—a further indication of low sensitivity to a Theory Y philosophy.

MOTIVATION AND NEEDS

The Need Hierarchy

There are five basic need systems according to Maslow, which can account for most of human behavior [61]. These needs are arranged in a hierarchy ranging from the most primitive and immature (with respect to the type behaviors they promote) to the most civilized and mature. Progression through this need hierarchy by a person may be thought of as roughly equivalent to climbing the rungs of a ladder, one at a time, where awareness of the next highest rung (and, consequently, the experiencing of a need to step up on it) is a function of having successfully negotiated the lower rung. Thus, the natural progression from need to need is thought to occur only to the extent that each lower need has, in turn, received adequate satisfaction.

Should satisfaction for a given need be blocked or unduly delayed, the individual will not develop any awareness of any higher need in the hierarchy; the lower the level at which this impairment occurs, the more primitive and immature are the behaviors employed likely to be. By the same token, should a need level eventually be negotiated after rather severe and prolonged deprivation, individuals may continue to be preoccupied with this need because it has never been—at least in their minds—completely or adequately satisfied; that is, they may become hypersensitive to that particular need.

Preoccupation with such lower need levels may predispose a person to revert back to those levels periodically, especially when higher order needs are blocked. This is a partial explanation of the classic response to frustration which is called regression, the adoption of less mature patterns of behavior under stressful conditions.

Unsatisfied Needs Affect Motivation

The strength of a given need is directly proportionate to its lack of satisfaction. Unsatisfied needs are strong sources of motivation, and satisfied needs yield little motivation. Similarly, since it is the un-

satisfied needs which make their presence felt, it will be these which determine the goals with which individuals are likely to be preoccupied and the goal-serving behaviors which they will employ. The significance of unsatisfied needs in the job setting, therefore, lies in the type of goals and goal-related behaviors which the needs evoke and the relevance of these, in turn, for the organization's program.

The Effect of Environment

There appears to be natural progression upward through the need hierarchy. When people become fixated at a lower level of motivation it is very likely because of constraints in their environment. One implication of this facet of motivation is that managers may be able to decide consciously whether they will function as a source of constraint or as a facilitator of higher level motives in their relationships. Too often, organizations and their representatives erect barriers to the natural progression and development, and either force people to regress to lower levels of motivation than they actually desire or arrest their development to such an extent that they learn to function at a level—typically low—which they perceive as appropriate if they are to remain in the organization. This suggests that the influence of the organization, and especially that of managers, may be as great or greater than that of an individual's personal makeup.

Job Structuring

In many respects, supervisors may be thought of as mediators of need satisfactions in the hospital; that is, they are the individuals who are likely to structure an employee's work in a particular way so that it lends itself to the use of certain behaviors which may be instrumental in attaining satisfaction of that person's needs. This means that the manner in which supervisors structure the work of their personnel has important implications for both the type of needs they will experience in their work and the likelihood that they will find satisfaction on the job.

The structuring of a job entails an analysis of the skills and needs of the worker, in addition to the more direct requirements of the job objectives per se, if truly high and constructive levels of employee motivation are to characterize their performance.

Management of Motives

Whether job designs will be rigid and concerned only with the nature of the end product, or whether they will also serve to create opportunities for the expression of employee needs is very much under the control of the supervisor. By the same token, supervisors' orientation to the whole issue of job design—whether they view it as a task with little latitude or as one of flexibility—will be significantly influenced by their personal "theory" of what makes people tick and how to motivate others. The nature of the job design—what it allows in the way of opportunities for need satisfaction—and the supervisors' personal theories about what motivates their employees are the two critical issues underlying the management of motives. It is these that will determine the extent to which a supervisor's employees will behave in mature and constructive ways in doing their work.

Should supervisors misread the needs of their employees and focus on inappropriate or irrelevant needs, their management will not have its desired effect. They will miss the target and find that their attempts to stimulate others have very little impact or, worse, unpredictable effects which create tension and a lack of cooperation.

EMPLOYEE NEEDS

Basic Needs

This need system reflects an individual's concern with comfort, strain avoidance, pleasant working conditions, and environmental supports. There may be a preoccupation with monetary rewards under this need, to the extent that they serve the achievement of comfort and material possessions in one's private or family affairs.

To the extent that employees are most motivated and stimulated by this need system, any job that serves this need is acceptable, and the nature of the work itself is relatively unimportant. When managers focus on this need system and emphasize it most in the management of others, they are acting on an assumption that people work primarily for monetary rewards and are concerned primarily with comfort, avoidance of fatigue, and the like. They will try to motivate others by offering wage increases, better working conditions, more leisure time, longer breaks, and administrative supports. In effect, they will try to motivate their employees to perform more effectively by emphasizing issues which are really unrelated to the nature of the work at hand.

The normal need strength is average at 48, but the supervisory personnel at the hospital had an average of 51, which indicates their basic needs are a bit higher than the norm and somewhat more unfilled, forcing the overemphasis of this need. (See Exhibit 1-11.)

Safety

This need system reflects an individual's concern with security and predictability. There is a need for order and assurance that one's job is secure and not subject to drastic change. In addition, there is a preoccupation

Exhibit 1-11. Comparison of Hospital Employee Needs and Maslow's Scale of Normative Values

Motivational Need	Need Strength Range		Average Need Strength	
	Normal	Hospital	Normal	Hospital
Basic	38–58	25–66	48	51
Safety	37–56	20–76	46	56
Belonging	43–63	34–98	54	60
Ego-status	64–84	44–89	75	65
Self-actualization	70–89	35–110	80	71

with fringe benefits of a protective nature, such as health insurance, worker compensation, and retirement income.

Individuals who are motivated by this kind of need system are those who value the job primarily as a defense against deprivation and loss of basic creature comfort satisfactions. This need system also involves issues which are peripheral to the work itself, and any job which affords safety, security, and long-range protections coupled with order and predictability will suffice.

If this is the salient need of the employees and managers focus on this need system in their management, managers will find that the employees respond in kind. That is, they will tend to meet the provisions of rules, regulations, job security, fringe benefits, and employee protections with fairly conforming and standardized performances. Little innovation or flexibility will be evidenced, risk taking will be avoided and employees will behave as good organization people.

While the normal high range for safety is 56, the high range at the hospital was 76, which corresponded to the high average score of 56 as compared with the normal need strength of 46. (See Exhibit 1-11.) The personnel indicated a serious lack of trust for the administration. They appeared to be preoccupied with security and motivated only to maintain what they are familiar with rather then developing positive, effective, alternative administrative strategies. Only limited innovation and limited risk taking can be expected until this need is fulfilled.

Belonging and Affiliation

This need system reflects an individual's concern with social relationships and a preoccupation with being an accepted member of the work group or of the organizational family. When this need is the primary source of motivation, individuals value their work as an opportunity for finding and establishing warm interpersonal relationships. Jobs which afford opportunities for a good deal of interaction with one's colleagues and bring one in contact with compatible people are likely to be valued, irrespective of their content.

Managers who identify this need system as the one of primary importance are likely to act in a particularly supportive and permissive way, while placing a good deal of emphasis on the activities of informal groups, extracurricular activities, such as organized sports programs and company picnics. The scale may be frequently tipped in favor of employees' personal and interpersonal objectives, if this will insure harmony and mutual acceptance. If such a need system is in fact the major source of motivation among one's employees, managerial emphasis of the need will lead to a fairly high level of employee satisfaction and loyalty, but this may be accompanied by a performance decrement since the individuals' attention may be diverted from work to social relationships—apparently with supervisory approval. At the same time, emphasis on this need system may often promote dependency and deter one's willingness to take dependent action or to risk alienation from the group, particularly where group performance issues are concerned.

While the normal high range is 63 with regard to the need to belong, the hospital supervisors had an actual high of 98, which was abnormally out of range, and this also corresponded to the high average score of 60 as compared with the normal need strength of 54. This need system of belongingness also relates to the last need system of security; the greater the need for safety, the greater the need to belong and be accepted as fulfillment. Work will give them this fulfillment but they are being forced to be overly supportive and permissive because of the current climate of uncertainty.

Ego-Status

This need system reflects an individual's concern with achieving special status in the work group or within an organization. As such it reflects a desire for recognition and for opportunities to demonstrate special competence; it is oriented essentially toward enhancement of the ego. It is the first need system discussed which is closely related to the nature of the work and dependent upon aspects of the job itself for satisfaction. Work which affords the opportunity to display those skills which individuals feel are important and in which they feel they are most competent will be valued as a means toward need satisfaction.

Managers who focus on this need system in their attempts to motivate others tend to emphasize public reward and recognition for services. To the extent that this need system is the dominant source of motivation among employees, a manager may promote both high morale and high performance rates by affording job designs which capitalize on the individual's need to excel, coupled with effective means of providing status-serving rewards.

The normal low range score for ego is at the level of 64, but the actual low score recorded for the hospital personnel was 44, which also corresponded to the low average score of 65 as compared with the normal need strength of 75. The respondents were not experiencing ego fulfillment with their work and appeared not to be optimally motivated to improve their intrinsic value, which was being inhibited by the increasing concern to fulfill safety needs and belongingness. When this need is unfulfilled, individuals will only seek to maintain their positions and not seek additional objectives, because of the high risk and uncertainty experienced and associated with failure and negative reward systems.

Self-Actualization

This need system reflects individuals' concern with testing their own potential, and involves a preoccupation with challenging opportunities and chances to be creative. The nature of the work is particularly critical to this need system, since in order for this source of motivation to be satisfied and continue to operate, the job must allow a good deal of control of fate, freedom of expression, and opportunities for experimentation. In effect, this need system, when it is dominant, motivates individuals to channel their most creative and constructive skills into their work.

Managers who focus primarily on this need system recognize that every job has areas within it which allow experimentation and innovation. When managers appropriately emphasize this need system, they are likely to find that both job satisfaction and performance surpass their expectations, for individual employees become partners in the enterprise as they seek to satisfy their own needs for expression and testing of potentials. Managers who emphasize this system are likely to use techniques for making work more meaningful; they may employ involvement strategies in planning job designs, make special assignments that capitalize on an individual's unique skills, or provide generous latitude to the employee group in fashioning work procedures and plans for implementation.

The normal low range score for self-actualization is at the level of 70, but the actual low score recorded for the supervisors was 35 (extremely low), which also corresponded to the low average score of 71 as compared with the normal need strength of 80.

Self-actualization is experienced when a supervisor "becomes everything he or she is capable of being." Many supervisors at the hospital will not attempt to self-actualize because their ego-status is much too low to risk this need fulfillment. Also, the previous low scores recorded on belonging and security account for the reluctance and trepidation felt by the supervisors. This leads to a protective climate and makes working less satisfying, less meaningful, and results in aborted goals and objectives.

The redesign of jobs is an essential component in rectifying this situation, which is temporary and can be corrected via future commitments on the part of top administra-

tion and a supportive climate where risk taking and creativity are encouraged and rewarded.

EMPLOYEE MOTIVATION AFFECTS LEADERSHIP

Maintenance Seekers

Those needs falling in the lower two and a half levels of the Maslow hierarchy (viz, basic, safety, and to a degree belongingness) are concerned with issues that are peripheral to the work. They involve a preoccupation with environmental factors and, rather than acting as sources of either true motivation or job satisfaction for an individual, they essentially concern hygienic aspects of the work.

When lower level needs are adequately satisfied, the work environment is clean in a psychological sense and does not interfere or compete with the job at hand. Satisfaction of such lower needs, however, will not bring about job satisfaction or increase work motivation. It simply alleviates dissatisfaction and frees individuals to become motivated if their work is rich enough in opportunities.

Attention to these lower need systems by management is primarily a maintenance function, which, if performed adequately, may prevent dissatisfactions. Although there are some individuals who derive their major orientations from these levels of needs, they are few in number. Those who do may be thought of primarily as maintenance seekers who will contribute little of a constructive nature to the hospital until they have been raised higher in the hierarchy of experienced needs. This is one of the functions of supervisors as they seek to motivate their employees.

Exhibit 1-12.   Profile of Hospital Employee Needs and Maslow's Scale of Normative Values

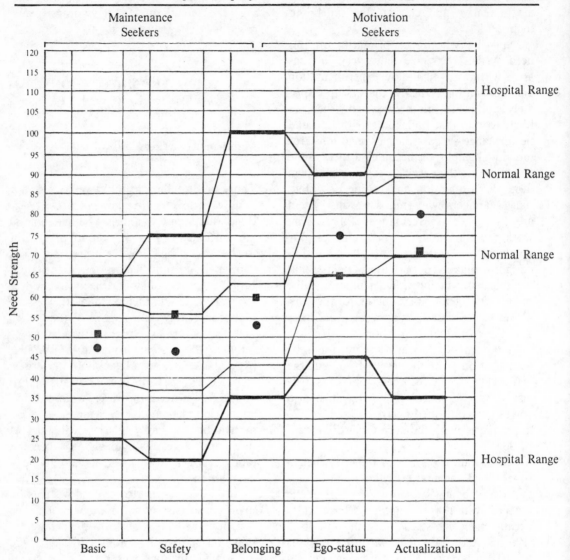

The hatched area represents the "average range" around those data points. Any departure of plots of ten or more points from this average range indicates a significant amount of either overemphasis or underemphasis of given needs depending on direction. Such deviations should be given considerable attention.

■ Normal Employees

● Hospital Employees

Motivation Seekers

The need for rewarding interpersonal relationships, opportunities to demonstrate special competence, and challenging enterprises which promote personal growth are the real sources of motivation in the work setting. Jobs can be designed in such a way as to provide opportunities for the satisfaction of such needs and, consequently, for the expression of those goal-directed behaviors which the hospital deems as truly motivated. Individuals with such higher level needs—and these far outnumber those at lower levels in the hierarchy—are thought of as motivation seekers.

To the extent that motivation seekers can find in their jobs attributes which afford and promote need satisfactions, they will tend to be motivated in a work sense and to experience job satisfaction. Supervisors who emphasize higher level needs help create motivation seekers and at the same time provide outlets for motivated behavior on the part of individuals who already operate at such higher levels. Supervisors mediate opportunities; they may either create barriers and frustrations for employees, or they may promote growth and create channels within the work for the expression of motivation-seeking behaviors. Exhibit 1-12 presents a profile of the need strengths of hospital and "normal" employees.

JOB SATISFACTION AFFECTS HOSPITAL GOALS

The need pattern and motivation of the hospital supervisors surveyed was at variance with normative behavior. The respondents' basic needs—the need for security and the need for belonging—were all greater than the normal range, which reflects their urgent concern with the climate of the hospital and changes being proposed and actualized by the current administration.

The needs usually associated with growth and development, namely ego-status and self-actualization, were both low, further reinforcing the fact that these individuals will not risk or invest in the hospital until they are more secure, supported, and included in decisions affecting their jobs and personal careers.

A resistive administrative climate discourages risk taking and creativity. Learning via management training and development will be stifled among employees who are overly concerned with meeting the basic needs, maintaining structure and functioning within a Theory X climate. If top administration indicates that the management development program is a current goal, then the best of efforts will be diluted within a closed climate.

A SYSTEMATIC APPROACH TO LEADERSHIP SELECTION

By Leo Plaszczynski, Jr.

Reprinted with permission from *The Journal of Nursing Administration*, Volume IX, Number 3, March 1979, pp. 7–15.

A system was developed at Burnham City Hospital, a 242-bed municipal general hospital in Champaign, Illinois, to aid in the selection of nursing leaders for all levels. It has been tested and refined over a four-year period with excellent results. Measures of certain leadership characteristics in an individual are converted into an objective score that is validated with independent subjective evaluation by a panel, measured against established criteria that any person aspiring to the position should meet. Advantages of this approach include a proven desire on the part of the applicant to be a leader, certification as a potential leader, peer competition, and an individual sense of achievement.

This system has been used to select nursing leaders at all levels including orderly, unit managers, head nurses, assistant head nurses, and nursing supervisors. The result is a strong group of leaders able to function in an environment of decentralized and participative management. The staff accepts the system as just and impartial. Those not selected but certified as potential leaders are encouraged to try again. Those not certified, but having a strong desire to lead, learn their specific shortcomings and attempt to correct them. The system has created not only good leaders but high morale and faith in nursing administration.

DESCRIPTION OF THE SYSTEM

The selection process includes five steps: application, objective assessment, subjective assessment, certification, and final selection. A description of the system follows.

Objective Assessment

In the objective assessment a relative value is assigned to the nine items considered in the application: nursing experience; length of service at our hospital; evaluations or references; previous leadership positions held; formal education; continuing education; major participation in projects, seminars, publications, and civic and academic affairs; and honors or awards. The total of these point values is recorded as the objective score.

The official application is the objective scoring sheet. (See Exhibit 1-13.)

An applicant must achieve a minimum objective score to become eligible to go before the panel. For each position a minimum acceptable value is assigned to each of the nine

Exhibit 1-13.   Objective Scoring Sheet for Clinical Promotion

NAME: _____ STATUS: _____ AGE: _____

POSITION APPLIED FOR:_____DATE:_____

1. Nursing experience in acute care facility:

    _____months full-time (1 point/month)   _____

    _____months part-time (1 point/month $X\frac{x}{5}$)   _____

2. Months employed at this hospital in any capacity:

    _____ (0.1 point/month)   _____

3. Performance evaluations or references:

    average (3)   above average (6)   outstanding (9)   _____

4. Leadership positions held: team leader (2)   assistant head nurse (4)

    head nurse (6)   supervisor (8)   other ( )   _____

5. Formal education: A.D.N. (60)   Diploma (90)   B.S.N. (120)

    Bachelor's Non-Nursing (108)   Master's Non-Nursing (135-162)

    M.S.N. (150-180)   Post-Graduate Nursing (1 point/credit)

    Post-Graduate Non-Nursing (0.9 points/credit)   _____

6. Continuing education (0.1 point/contact hour)   _____

7. Committee participation: member (0.1 CH × 10 mos/year)   _____

    office (0.15 CH × 10 mos/year)   _____

    chairperson (0.2 CH × 10 mos/yr.)   _____

8. Major participations: seminars, workshops, inservice   _____

    publications   _____

    civic   _____

    academic   _____

9. Awards, honors: academic   _____

    civic   _____

    professional   _____

TOTAL   _____

PANEL   _____

CERTIFIED: YES   NO   _____

items and totaled for a minimum score. The job description for a particular position mandates values for some of the items. For example, if the position of head nurse requires three years' experience as a staff nurse, applicants for the head nurse position need a minimum of 36 points for the nursing experience item.

Scoring. To assist the nurse administrator in completing the objective assessment, scoring guidelines are provided. (See Exhibit 1-14.)

The first item we consider is nursing experience. Only experience directly related to

our type of facility is counted. For example, since our medical-surgical hospital has no psychiatric or rehabilitative wards, we would not award experience credit in these areas. Experience in office, clinic, and public health nursing is not directly related, so we award no credit. In the case of nursing educators, we must assess how much exposure they have had to basic medical-surgical clinical practice. If we are looking for an inservice coordinator, all the educator's experience would be counted. The value assigned is one point for every month of full-time experience. For part-time

Exhibit 1-14. Scoring Objective Scoring Sheet for Clinical Promotion

Purpose: To ascertain an applicant's eligibility for promotion in accordance with the job description requirements.

Special instructions:

Regardless of overall score, the applicant must have the appropriate number of points on the following items:

1. Nursing care in acute care facility.
2. Performance evaluations or references.
3. Leadership position(s) held.
4. Formal education (the diploma or degree must be from an accredited school or college of nursing).

Procedure:

STEPS	EXPLANATION
1. Enter complete name of applicant.	1. Last name, first name, and middle initial.
2. Enter current position of applicant.	2. Team leader, assistant head nurse, head nurse, coordinator.
3. Enter age of applicant.	3. As of the last birthday.
4. Enter position for which applicant has applied.	4. Include specific unit or division.
5. Enter date.	5. Use date objective scoring sheet is being initiated.
6. Complete all scoring items.	6.
A. Items which have a pre-determined value.	
1) Enter nursing experience in an acute care medical-surgical facility.	1) a. Score one point for each month of full-time experience.
	b. Score one point times days per week worked divided by 20 for part-time experience.
	c. Only experience on medical-surgical service and inservice in acute care facility should be counted.
	d. Experience in a nursing home, extended care facility, or convalescent center can be counted if the facility is known to have maximum care beds.
	e. Exclude experience in psychiatry, public health, office, educational, industrial, or clinic nursing.
	f. If the applicant performed full-time medical-surgical patient care duties in an excluded area, it may be counted, i.e., surgical ward of a psychiatric hospital.

Exhibit 1-14. continued

STEPS	EXPLANATION
2) Enter number of months employed at the hospital in any capacity.	2) This awards the applicant credit for loyalty and service to the hospital. a. Score one-tenth of a point for each month served whether full-time or part-time. b. Give credit for all positions held (i.e., messenger, orderly, nursing unit secretary).
3) Review performance evaluations or reference ratings.	3) Score the appropriate points which were set up on a relative scale. a. If the applicant has three or more evaluations at this hospital, use only these. b. If the applicant has fewer than three, use references from other employers as well as the evaluations to determine scores. c. If there are numerous evaluations and the last three have progressively improved, use only these three to determine score.
4) Review all leadership positions held.	4) Add the scores for each position held and enter total in scoring column. "Other" may be a unique leadership position for which the scorer may assign a value or refer it to the panel for assignment of value. Scoring is relative; i.e., each institution can decide on the number of points assignable to any position.
6. A. 5) Review the appropriate formal education completed.	5) Score the appropriate number of points, on the basis of one point per credit. This is derived from the established system of continuing education units awarded for continuing education. One CEU = 10 contact hours times $0.1 = 1$. a. Assuming an associate degree nursing program is four full semesters in which 60 credits are earned in 600 contact hours, 600 hours times $0.1 = 60$ points = 60 semester credits. b. The diploma school is assumed to be six semesters (90 points). c. Baccalaureate degrees outside of nursing and nursing education have a value slightly less than a BSN and are calculated at 0.9 points per credit. d. Masters' programs vary in length from one to two years; therefore, credits can vary from 30 to 60. If the job requires a completed master's degree, then the point requirement will vary with the number of credits needed for a completed program. (For a one-year completed master's program points for

Exhibit 1-14. continued

STEPS	EXPLANATION
	eight baccalaureate semesters and two master's semesters are required, total 150. For a two-year master's program, 180.)
	e. Credits earned prior to baccalaureate completion or postbaccalaureate or postgraduate can be scored by assigning one point per semester credit earned. Non-nursing related credits would earn 0.9 per semester credit.
6) List continuing education.	6) All listed continuing education should be verified by a certificate, letter from education department, or travel voucher.
	a. Score 0.1 for each contact hour, excluding breaks, meals, etc.
	b. Total points for each program and enter in scoring column.
	c. All continuing education programs must be directly or indirectly related to nursing. The panel shall rule on eligible programs.
7) List membership on committees, professional organizations (length of membership and offices held) on back of sheet.	7) Reasonable proof of membership or offices held should be supplied. Attendance at meetings should be considered.
	a. Award 0.1 for each contact hour of meeting for a maximum of ten months out of the year. Example: if the applicant was a committee member for one year and met once a month for two hours, the maximum points given would be two hours times ten months = 20 hours times 0.1 per hour = two points.
	b. Award 0.15 in the same manner as above if the applicant held an office other than chairperson.
	c. Award 0.2 points, as above, for each contact hour served as chairperson.
8) List all major participations on the back for:	8) Points may be awarded by the scorer or the panel in one of two ways: based on a relative scale, probably 1–10; or based on estimated contact hours involved.
a. seminars, workshops, inservice	a. Participation in seminars, workshops, and inservice where the applicant prepared, organized, and presented material as a lecturer or group leader.
b. publications	b. Publication on a subject related to nursing in a recognized journal or trade magazine.
c. civic	c. Participation in a civic program related to nursing, such as public education on cancer or arthritis; service on a government committee or task force relating to the health field in which an acute care hospital would be involved.
d. academic	d. Academic is defined as serving as a guest lecturer, instructor, or advisor in a higher education setting.

Exhibit 1-14. continued

STEPS	EXPLANATION
6. A. 9) List all awards and total score for following achievements:	9) Awards and honors should be recognized as an achievement gained by outstanding performance.
a. academic	a. Scholarships or certificates for outstanding scholastic achievements, for which there was competition among the student populace.
b. civic	b. Recognition of civic awards should be selective and limited to a few (e.g., outstanding citizen award).
c. professional	c. Professional awards must be limited to those conferred by a recognized group within the applicant's area of practice.
B. Total score sheet to determine eligibility for paneling.	B. 1) This may be delayed if panel is to assign values for items 7–9; however, if scores for the required elements are met and if eligibility could be determined without items 7–9, then paneling should be scheduled using a tentative total score.
	2) It may be necessary to schedule an interview with the applicant to substantiate items 7–9.
7. Schedule applicant for panel.	

work, a comparable value is assigned, based on the number of days' experience per week.

We wished to give some recognition to loyal service and seniority in our hospital, so our second element was credit for months employed at Burnham City Hospital in any capacity. However, we did not want this element to outweigh the others, since it would be important only when all other things were fairly equal between two or more candidates. Thus, we assigned to seniority a value of only one-tenth the experience value.

Unlike the experience element, this element is not required in the job description and it is not figured in calculating the minimum objective score.

How should points be awarded for performance evaluations? This was a difficult question and we could not find any objective basis for assigning value. As a result, we had to rely on a relative assignment. We felt justified in using relative values since all candidates would be assessed on the same scale, which makes the score a comparative valua-

tion of candidates measured against predetermined established criteria. For in-house candidates we decided to assign three points to the average performance rating, six to the above average, and nine to the outstanding or excellent, based on the last three performance evaluations.

If an insufficient number of evaluations were available, or if the candidate was an outside applicant, we assigned values to the reference ratings supplied by former employers.

Each job description states the required performance rating for the position. Because we prefer our head nurses to be above average, that is the required performance rating for the position. In lesser positions, an average rating may be sufficient.

Leadership positions held is another item that had to be assigned a relative value. Score requirements for this item can vary, but the required score should be stated in the job description—for example, experience as an assistant head nurse (4 points) is required of all candidates for a head nurse position. A score below four would exclude the candidate from consideration. Different institutions use various titles for both staff and line leaders. Thus, the scorer must try to determine the level of an outsider's position vis-a-vis our structure and, in the "other" block, assign a value to the title.

Formal education is easy to assess. Allowance is made for indirectly related credits, but credits directly related to a nursing degree are emphasized. Therefore, 0.9 is given for non-nursing credits whereas a whole point is given for nursing credits.

The next element, continuing education, is assessed on the basis of the contact hour. The problem is in determining whether the subject matter for which the contact hours have been earned is applicable to nursing. We accept and score equally all subject matter, whether directly or indirectly related to nursing.

Nursing leaders should be involved in the profession, and so we expect certain candidates to have served on committees. These committees may be in the hospital, the professional organization, or the community. All are a source of experience and learning, provided they are related to nursing or leadership. Holding an office or chairing a committee requires greater participation and confers more experience; hence, these activities increase the score slightly.

If the job requirement calls for participation on committees and extensive continuing education, the candidate must have a certain number of points for each of these items. For example, a head nurse might be required to have a minimum of three points for committee participation and six points for continuing education.

An element also valued highly in our institution is "major participation" in four areas; 1) seminars, workshops, and inservice; 2) publications; 3) civic affairs; 4) academic affairs. Scores for this item are given largely on a subjective basis by the scorer or the entire panel, but the contact hour system can be used to some extent.

Major participation in seminars, workshops, and inservice is defined as having a major role as organizer, speaker, or educator in any of these activities.

Publishing an article or book related to nursing attests to the professional's desire to inform colleagues of new ideas or opinions and should be highly valued. A scale might be set up by which the candidate would receive points according to the worth of the article or book. The panel could be asked to participate in assessing the publication and assigning a score.

Civic participation can be defined as participation in any program that educates the public in an area of nursing or health care in which the candidate has expertise. A nurse who holds prenatal lectures for expectant parents would be given credit. One who serves on a civic committee to determine the community's needs for health resources is given credit. Either independent criteria or the contact hour can be used for scoring.

Many nurses are asked to serve as guest lecturers, advisory committee members, and planners for schools and colleges of nursing. Again, candidates are awarded a score for such participation.

The final item on our objective scoring sheet is awards and honors. These are broken down into three categories: academic, civic, and professional. Academic awards and honors earned through scholastic achievements are assigned a relative value by the scorer or panel.

Civic and professional awards are given in recognition of a major contribution to the community or profession; for example, a nurse may be honored by the Jaycees for her role in establishing downtown health centers, or she may be chosen as the outstanding member of the year by her nursing association.

In most cases, neither major participation nor honors are job requirements; nevertheless, they increase the candidate's certifying score, provided she has met all the required scores. If an involved and participative leader is sought, these items should be given strong consideration.

Subjective Assessment

The subjective assessment is performed through a series of carefully designed questions, usually situational, which the candidate is expected to answer spontaneously but fully.

Choosing the assessment panel. An important consideration arises immediately: who should perform this subjective assessment? In our hospital a panel of four raters works well. This number is sufficient to allow varying opinions and yet permits consensus through minimal discussion. Any prejudice or bias can readily be identified.

Leaders should select leaders, especially if they are responsible and accountable for the new leader's performance. To select our panel, we begin with the predecessor, if possible, and go up the organizational structure and command chain to the chief executive officer, if necessary. To introduce a different perspective, we select as one panel member a department head from outside the nursing department. A physician may be desirable on the panel. Since they are judging for leadership and not clinical practice, non-nurses and nurses have rendered remarkably similar ratings over the past four years. In fact, the highest and lowest ratings usually vary by less than ten points.

Selecting the right members for the panel is the job of the nursing director. When the person vacating the position has proven to be a good leader, it is wise to provide a replacement attuned to her philosophies and beliefs. The most important member of the panel is the person to whom the successful candidate will report directly.

Often, the predecessor and immediate supervisor may come to the panel with prejudices for or against a candidate they know well. It is surprising how quickly this prejudice is eliminated or minimized by the objective attitude of the rest of the panel. Although some prejudice occasionally filters through, it can be reconciled in the scoring procedure.

Designing and testing the questions. The design of the panel questions is very important. Questions should measure knowledge, reaction, communication skills, common sense, and mental process. There should be a good, better, and best answer to each question.

In Exhibit 1-15, 14 areas and sample questions are listed for consideration. It is not necessary to examine candidates on all 14 areas. Questions must be worded in such a manner that the applicant is led directly to the right track. Questions that can be answered in just a few words should be avoided. Though specific information is being elicited, there must be room for broad, general answers. The candidate's personal philosophy and experiences should influence the answers.

Situational questions are the most revealing. A question beginning, "What would you do if . . ." will measure the individual's ability to think in the face of a stressful situation. A question beginning, "Why do you think that . . . " is designed to elicit an opinion. To measure a person's basic knowledge, it is best to ask a question whose answer would include many basic single-word characteristics (for example, "What are some of the basic characteristics of a good leader?")

Fourteen areas are listed in Exhibit 1-15, but the reader certainly can think of many more. It is recommended that several series of questions be designed in each area so that candidates will never know beforehand the precise questions to be asked. However, the areas on which candidates are examined are

Exhibit 1-15.   Guide for Designing Panel Questions

Though panel questions should measure the candidate's basic knowledge of leadership principles, they are designed primarily to measure the candidate's ability to make decisions under stress. Given a minimum of facts in a situational question, the candidate should give not a right or wrong answer, but an acceptable answer that will most likely resolve the situation. Often, there are many ways to resolve a situation, so the candidate is given the opportunity to be original and innovative.

Even with questions that test basic knowledge, there is room for a good, better, or best answer (for example, "Describe in detail, what you would do if you were assigned to plan and present an inservice program.") Here, as in other questions, we look for the anatomy of a principle. Anatomy varies and so will the answers, but they will be recognizable when compared to the model.

It is recommended that both situational and basic knowledge questions be developed in the following areas:

AREA	SAMPLE QUESTION
1. Organizational structure	1. In your present position, can you give the names of all those above you, from your immediate supervisor to the chief executive officer?
2. Problem solving	2. In your own words, can you identify the five basic steps of problem solving?
3. Discipline	3. What would you do if a nurse refused assignment?
4. Policy resources	4. Where would you find resources on isolation?
5. Public relations	5. How would you handle a visitor who refused to leave after normal visiting hours?
6. Staffing resources	6. At the last minute, a night charge nurse calls in and you have no replacement. How would you handle it?
7. Planning, organizing, and implementing education.	7. The new intracranial pressure monitor has arrived and you have been assigned the responsibility of inservicing it. How would you go about it?
8. Stress problem resolution	8. A physician has just screamed at the charge nurse and she has quit on the spot. What would you do?
9. Proposals	9. You have struck upon an innovation that will save time and money. What elements should be contained in your written proposal?
10. Clinical intervention	10. You see a nurse about to do something not in accordance with procedure. What steps would you take, and when?
11. Delegating	11. You have five projects all due on the same day and not enough time to do them. What can you do about it?
12. Evaluating employee or situation or equipment	12. You have been assigned a project of evaluating a new syringe. How would you gather your information for the evaluation?
13. Counseling	13. Jane Doe is making many mistakes, which is unlike her. How would you counsel her?
14. Legal	14. While looking up something in the State Hospital Regulations, you discover a violation in practice. What would you do?

There are many alternatives to these sample questions, and there are many other questions that can be asked. These questions and answers are designed not to render an absolute score, but to serve as a guide for the panel members to rate candidates on how they respond, what they respond, and the efficacy of the answer. Is it a good answer? Is it better than average; is it the best they have heard?

identical so that results can be statistically measured and compared. For example, one set of candidates might be asked, "What are the five basic steps of problem solving?"; the next set could be asked, "If you have a problem, what steps would you take to solve it?"

Panel members can be assisted by providing them a "cheat" sheet containing appropriate elements that would constitute answers for some questions. They can then rate candidates better by determining the number and quality of these elements in the candidate's answer.

Often a candidate gives a good answer, but one that is completely off the desired track. Panel members quickly sense whether the person might better answer the question if it was redirected. It is the chairperson's responsibility to restate the question carefully without supplying additional information that would give the candidate an advantage over the others. If a question is redirected to an early candidate the panel may ask the question both ways for subsequent candidates.

To make sure that questions are worded to elicit the desired answers, test them on established leaders by asking them of several supervisors on your staff. If the questions elicit off-track answers, they should be revised.

Testing the questions will identify certain nouns or adjectives that may be included on the panel members' "cheat" sheet. Each question can be validated by use of some statistical formula. In over four years of using the system, our sample questions have been well tested and revised where necessary.

We have found that ten questions elicit sufficient information, but any number can be asked and the required subjective score adjusted accordingly. In the first nine questions we have tried to cover as many areas as possible. The tenth question serves a special purpose, explained later. Once the panel has been selected and oriented, and a set of valid and appropriate questions designed, the subjective assessment may be conducted. Exhibit 1-16 outlines the procedure for doing so, beginning with initial briefing about the candidates' objective assessment.

Rating and tallying. The first nine answers are rated on a scale from zero to ten, with five being considered the middle, or average. Each answer is rated individually by each panel member. The tenth item is, in fact, not a question but a subjective overall rating that considers the candidate's answers, delivery, conduct, posture, logic, and other elements commonly considered in judging a first impression. Panel members attempt to rank the individual in comparison to the ideal candidate, not to the other candidates.

When the interview is completed, and the candidate dismissed, the panel members tally their ratings to arrive at their individual scores. Discussion is discouraged until the chairperson receives the four totaled scores. The scores are then added together and divided by four to determine the total subjective score. In our experience, the difference between the lowest and the highest of four individual scores has been less than 10 or 12 points. This has become our acceptable range of variance. If the variance is greater, this is a cue that either an arithmetical miscalculation or bias has occurred. Rechecking the arithmetic is simple; dealing with bias is much more difficult. If one member consistently marked higher or lower than the others, his bias becomes obvious. Sometimes the score difference on a single question may be the cause of an unacceptable variance. Each member's score sheet is then returned and ratings are compared, question by question. The panel engages in a discussion, and the high or low rater is given the opportunity to re-rate the answer to the particular question, though he is under no

Exhibit 1-16.   Conducting the Subjective Assessment

STEPS	EXPLANATION
1. Brief members as to candidate's objective scoring sheet and resume.	1. Panel should assign any point values for items on the scoring sheet left to their discretion, (i.e., awards, honors, major project participation). This step may be delayed until after the interview if the panel is not to have the background information beforehand.
2. Adjust objective score.	2. Again, this may be delayed until after the interview.
3. Review sheet of selected questions.	3. To help panel evaluate answers expected and assign a value.
4. Present candidate to panel.	4. Introduce panel to candidate using full name and title: a. Handshaking is in order. b. Place candidate at a distance from panel so rating can be done confidentially and comfortably.
5. If no resume was submitted, ask candidate to tell a little about herself.	5. Candidate should include background, schooling, work experience, future goals, and why she applied for this position.
6. Give candidate questions to study for three to five minutes.	6. Each panel member should have an individual scoring sheet entering the candidate's name and position applied for. Each listed question has a scoring scale from 0-10 with five being considered average or satisfactory.
7. The chairperson will ask the questions one at a time.	7. A reasonable time should be allowed for a complete answer. Any clarification of the questions should be done only by the chairperson and should be repeated to all ensuing candidates. Sometimes the answer may go off in a wrong direction, and the chairperson may have to redirect the question.
8. Invite panel members to ask questions.	8. Any question may be asked that will help assign an overall rating to the candidate.
9. Invite the candidate to question the panel.	9. Every attempt should be made to give honest answers.
10. Dismiss candidate.	10. Thank the candidate for appearing and give an indication when the results will be forthcoming.
11. Repeat steps 1–10 for each candidate.	

obligation to do so. The consistently high or low rater is given the opportunity to adjust his total score to fall within the 10–12 point range of variance. The entire panel must agree on the subjective score before it can be used to certify a candidate.

Each position requires a minimum subjective score, with higher level positions requiring higher subjective scores. The following is a list of minimum acceptable subjective scores:

Assistant Head Nurse; Nurse Specialist	50
Head Nurse; Nurse Clinician	55
Coordinator; Clinical Specialist	60
Assistant Director	70

Certifying the Candidate

If the subjective score meets the minimum required for the position it is then taken together with the objective score. The objective score is rechecked to see that each requirement in the job description has been met. The two scores are added to obtain the certifying score, which must meet a minimum for each position. Following are the total scores (objective plus subjective) required for certification for a number of positions:

Assistant Head Nurse	125 (75 + 50)
Head Nurse	140 (85 + 55)
Nurse Specialist	170 (120 + 50)
Nurse Clinician	235 (180 + 55)
Clinical Specialist	245 to 275 (185 to 215 + 60)
Division or Shift Coordinator	185 (125 + 60)
Inservice Coordinator	245 (185 + 60)
Assistant Director	215 (145 + 70)

Through this process, each candidate's qualifications are converted to numerical values to facilitate comparison with other candidates and to determine if all the minimum requirements have been satisfied. Once certified for a position, the candidate remains certified for a position at that level only. However, a staff nurse who certifies for a head nurse position but is not selected, is meeting or exceeding the requirements for an assistant head nurse position and can be considered certified for it without paneling.

Whether a candidate is successful or not, she can be told exactly where she stood vis-a-vis requirements and other candidates.

The Final Selection

The final step in the process is adapted from an approach used by the Civil Service Commission. The commission makes more than one candidate eligible for selection by a panel. If three or more candidates certify, we eliminate all but the top two. The same panel chosen to conduct the subjective assessment selects the top two candidates and, finally, the top candidate.

Background information about the candidates is reviewed again and the panel discusses every aspect of the objective and subjective assessment. The chairperson then calls for a vote, which may be verbal or written. In the event of a tie, ensuing votes are by secret ballot because someone must compromise, and the secret ballot is a face-saver.

Panel members are instructed not to discuss the proceedings. Unsuccessful candidates are contacted by the chairperson as soon as possible and notified of their ranking. They are counseled on their deficits, and encouraged on their strengths. Should the top candidate decide to reject the position, the second best candidate is in line to receive the offer.

Unsuccessful candidates who have been certified may apply for future vacancies without going before the panel again. Their objective score is updated, but their subjective score is used again and added to the new objective score. The candidate may opt to go before the panel again in the hope of improving her subjective score.

Once the candidate accepts the position, we have a new leader who has been chosen on her merits, her input, her preparation, and her aspirations. The chance of poor performance is remote. In our experience in four years, only one selected head nurse candidate has turned out to be ineffective in her position. Some nurses selected for lower leadership positions did not fare as well. Yet, out of some 80 to 100 positions filled through this system, fewer than 5 percent were filled by candidates who proved less than desirable for one reason or another. In most of these cases, the deficiency was probably due to unstable conditions in the individual's personal life; however, we have not undertaken any study to prove this.

REACTION TO THE SYSTEM

Administration. Both nursing and hospital administrators readily accepted this system because it provided a tool that guaranteed a close look at persons who would play an important role in determining the direction the institution would take. Such participation in the selection process is in keeping with the philosophy of participative management.

Staff. In many surveys, employees rate fairness as an important attribute of a good job. This promotional system is unanimously rated as fair by our staff. They consider it tough and stressful, but as equitable as is possible. Confidence in management is restored and an offer of a management position is highly regarded. Staff members who recognize their shortcomings never bother to apply. When no candidates from within the organization are acceptable, the successful outside candidate is quickly accepted as an expert in her area. There is a genuine feeling that each person has a chance for promotion provided she meets the minimum requirements and is the best among competing peers. In addition the new leader is more quickly accepted by the staff because of their respect for one or more of the panelists.

Individual. The candidate who has undergone a paneling or even an unacceptable application experiences stress. She is counseled regarding her deficits, or weaknesses, and is advised on what is needed to correct them. The failing candidate does not internalize the blame nor externalize it by blaming a supervisor. Because objective reasons for failure are identified which are often correctable, promotion remains possible.

FILLING IN THE MATRIX: LEADERSHIP THEORIES

The model being used in this anthology represents a matrix in which the leader is placed in an environment. Many theories and concepts presented in this section can be used as you fill out the matrix presented in the model. Leadership theories can be correlated with the model as you consider your own concepts of leadership.

1. Central to the model is the leader. Leadership theories that focus on the leader include the "great man" theory and the trait theories of leadership. Using this model, consider your own leadership development.

a. How have the events in your personal life influenced your leadership development? Are the traits that you have developed a function of your genetic heritage, of your childhood, or of your school experience?

b. How has the profession of nursing influenced your leadership development? Consider the influence of your first nursing education program, of your first position as a registered nurse, of the major events in your education and work experience as a professional.

c. How does your personal life now influence your leadership development? Are you supported by your family and friends? Are there factors in your personal life that encourage your motivation for leadership? Are there factors in your personal life that serve as barriers to your leadership?

d. After considering your leadership development, do you support the theory that certain people become leaders because they are unique? Does your experience support the theory that leaders have certain traits that enable them to be leaders?

2. As we move from the circle of the leader in the central part of our model, we introduce variables of home, family, community, social sanction, and the health care industry. These variables imply that leaders function in groups; leadership theories that apply to these sections of the model include the group theories, which explain leadership as an exchange between leaders and followers, situation theories, which include designations of favorable and unfavorable situations, and the path-goal theory, which describes leadership behaviors as supportive, directive, participative, and achievement-oriented.

   a. Which of these theories appeals to you as being most relevant to your own perception of leadership?

   b. As a leader in your work, do you function mainly in group exchanges with those you lead? Or, do you perceive yourself as dealing with and in situations? Is your current situation favorable or unfavorable for your leadership? Do you see yourself as leading others toward goals through your leadership? If so, are you directive, supportive, participative, or achievement-oriented?

   c. If you selected one of the four types of leadership styles—directive, supportive, participative, or achievement-oriented—consider your basis for the selection:

   i. Did you select the style because of your own leadership style or your personal traits?

   ii. Did you select the style because of the competencies and abilities of those whom you lead?

   iii. Did you select the style because of the nature of the work that you are responsible for accomplishing through your leadership?

3. Other leadership theories that fit into our model include Likert's four systems; McGregor's Theory X, Theory Y; and Reddin's three-dimensional model. These theories and models suggest that interaction is a primary component of leadership. The variables considered by Likert to be intervening variables in determining leadership behaviors are listed below for your consideration of these interaction theories.

   a. How do you interact with those you lead in terms of:

   i. Communication

   ii. Influence

   iii. Responsibility

   iv. Motivation

   v. Coordination

   vi. Decision making

   b. Do your responses give you cues as to the style of leadership you use?

4. The Vroom-Yetton model focuses on the leader's decision making. This model encompasses all components of the model used in our anthology in that the leader uses information from the immediate and from the more distant environmental forces shown as the outermost rings in the model.

   a. Do you think that decision making is the central focus of your leadership?

   b. When you evaluate other leaders, is their decision-making ability a major factor in whether you consider them to be successful or unsuccessful?

5. Applebaum discusses leadership in terms of differences in open and closed climates.

a. Consider the climate in which you work; is it open? Is it closed? Is your style like that of most of the other leaders? What leadership styles are rewarded?

b. Internal and external locus of control are mentioned in both Heinmann's and Applebaum's articles. Consider your own behavior: do you require much external control? Are those you lead dependent on external control from you? Do you adjust the amount of external control that you give to those you lead according to their needs?

c. Of the following factors, some may be more important to you than others in explaining why you have the position you now hold. Rate the items from 1 to 5, assigning a 1 to those of the highest importance to you.

_____*The amount of money earned*

_____*The degree of autonomy that you have*

_____*The ability to give directions to others, to be boss*

_____*The ability to accomplish important and meaningful goals*

_____*The degree of comfort and convenience in the job*

d. Your response to the rating may indicate some of the features of your position that are important to you. Consider how the following, mentioned by Applebaum, influence your leadership:

  i. Job structure
  ii. Meeting your basic needs
  iii. Your level of motivation
  iv. Your need to maintain your status

e. Because there is no universally accepted theory of leadership, you may wish to integrate many theories into one of your own. How do you describe your own framework of leadership?

REFERENCES AND NOTES

1. All specific references made to the styles-of-leadership study are drawn from Lewin, K., Lippitt, R., and White, R. K. Patterns of aggressive behavior in experimentally created "social climates," **J. Social Psychol.**, pp. 271–276, May, 1939.
2. Lewin, K., Lippitt, R., and White, R. K., 1939, p. 284.
3. Lewin, K., Lippitt, R., and White, R. K., 1939, p. 284.
4. Stogdill, R. M., and Coons, A. E. (Eds.), **Leader Behavior: Its Description and Measurement,** Columbus: Bureau of Business Research, Ohio State University, 1957.
5. Stogdill, R. M., and Coons, A. E., 1957, pp. 42–43.
6. Likert, R. Foreword. In Katz, D., Maccoby, and Morse, N. C. **Productivity, Supervision and Morale in an Office Situation.** Ann Arbor: Survey Research Center, University of Michigan, 1950.
7. Likert, R., 1950, p. 62.
8. Likert, R., **New Patterns of Management,** New York: McGraw-Hill, 1961.
9. Davis, K. **Human Behavior at Work** (4th ed.) New York: McGraw-Hill, 1972, pp. 103–104.
10. Hollander, E. P., and Julian, J. W. Contemporary trends in the analysis of leadership processes. **Psychol. Bull.**, 71:387–397, 1969. Reprinted in Steers, R. M., and Porter, L. W. (Eds.) **Motivation and Work Behavior.** New York: McGraw-Hill, 1975, p. 349.
11. Filley, A. C., House, R. J., and Kerr, S. **Managerial Process and Organizational Behavior** (2nd ed.) Glenview, Ill.: Scott, Foresman, 1976, pp. 219–222.
12. See Greene, C. N., A longitudinal analysis of relationships among leader behavior and subordinate performance and satisfaction, **Academy of Management Proceedings,** pp. 433–440, 1973, and Kerr, S., and Schriesheim, C., Consideration, initiating structure and organizational criteria: an update of Korman's 1966 review, **Personnel Psychol.**, pp. 555–568, Winter, 1974.
13. Fiedler, F. E. **A Theory of Leadership Effectiveness.** New York: McGraw-Hill, 1967, pp. 143–144.
14. Fiedler, F. E., 1967, p. 147.
15. Fiedler, F. E., 1967, p. 147.
16. Fiedler, F., and Chemers, M. M. **Leadership and Effective Management.** Glenview, Ill.: Scott, Foresman, 1974, p. 83.
17. Fiedler, F. E. Engineer the job to fit the manager. **Harvard Business Rev.**, pp. 115–122, Sept.–Oct., 1965.
18. Filley, A. C., House, R. J., and Kerr, S., 1976, p. 261.
19. See Luthans, F., **Introduction to Management: A Contingency Approach,** New York: McGraw-Hill, 1976, for a contingency framework for management as a whole.
20. Georgopoulos, B. S., Mahoney, G. M., and Jones, N. W. A path-goal approach to productivity. **J. Appl. Psychol.**, pp. 345–353, Dec., 1957. Evans, M. G. The effect of supervisory behavior on the path-goal relationship. **Organizational Behavior and Human Performance,** pp. 277–298, May, 1970; and House, R. J. A path-goal theory of leader effectiveness. **Administrative Sci. Quart.**, pp. 321–338, Sept., 1971.
21. House, R. J., and Mitchell, T. R. Path-goal theory of leadership. **J. Contemp. Business,** pp. 81–97, Autumn, 1974.
22. House, R. J., and Mitchell, T. R., 1974, pp. 81–97.
23. House, R. J, and Mitchell, T. R., in Steers, R. M., and Porter, L. W., 1975, p. 386.
24. Filley, A. C., House, R. J., and Kerr, S., 1976, p. 254.
25. House, R. J., and Mitchell, T. R., in Steers, R. M., and Porter, L. W., 1975, pp. 385–386.
26. Filley, A. C., House, R. J., and Kerr, S., 1976, pp. 256–260.

27. Reddin, W. J. Managing organizational change. **Personnel J.**, p. 503, July, 1969.
28. Likert, R. **The Human Organization**. New York: McGraw-Hill, 1967., pp. 3, 11.
29. Likert, R., 1967, pp. 26, 29.
30. Likert, R., 1967, pp. 80–81.
31. Webb, E. J., et. al. **Unobtrusive Measures Nonreactive Research in the Social Sciences**. Chicago: Rand McNally, 1966.
32. Likert, R., 1967, p. 192.
33. Vroom, V. H., and Yetton, P. W. **Leadership and Decision-Making**. Pittsburgh: University of Pittsburgh Press, 1973, chap. 3.
34. Vroom, V. H. A new look at managerial decision making. **Organizational Dynamics** 1(4): 77, 1973.
35. Hagen, E., and Wolff, L. **Nursing Leadership Behavior in General Hospitals**. New York: Teachers College, Columbia University, 1961, p. 6.
36. Hagen, E., and Wolff, L., 1961, p. 18.
37. Fiedler, F. E., 1967, p. 8.
38. Fiedler, F. E., 1967, p. 11.
39. Eggers, E. T. The essence of leadership. **Super. Nurse**, 3:23, Dec., 1972.
40. Keaveny, M. E. Leadership: what is it: **Super. Nurse**, 4:30 ff., 1970.
41. Kelber, M. Accent on leadership. **Internat. Nurs. Rev.**, 7:5, 1970.
42. Argyris, C. **Personality and Organization**. New York: Harper and Brothers, 1957, p. 211.
43. Tead, O. **The Art of Leadership**. New York: McGraw-Hill, 1935.
44. Argyris, C., 1957, pp. 129–130.
45. Argyris, C., 1957, p. 189.
46. Argyris, C., 1957, p. 192.
47. Uris, A. **Techniques of Leadership**. New York: McGraw-Hill, 1953, p. 31.
48. Bernard, L.L. **An Introduction to Social Psychology**. New York: Henry Holt, 1926.
49. Bernard, L. L., 1926, pp. 528–540.
50. Tead, O., 1935.
51. Tead, O., 1935, pp. 82–151, 257–266.
52. Brown, J. F. **Psychology and the Social Order**. New York: McGraw-Hill, 1936, p. 331.
53. Brown, J. F., 1936, p. 331.
54. Slaughter, F. G. **Immortal Magyar Semmelweis, Conqueror of Childbed Fever**. New York: Henry Schuman, 1950.
55. Gibb. C. A. The principles and traits of leadership. **J. Abnorm. Social Psychol.** 42:901, 1947.
56. Brown, J. F., 1936.
57. Brown, J. F., 1936, chap. 17.
58. Stogdill, R. M. **Handbook of Leadership**. New York: Free Press, 1974.
59. McGregor, D. **The Human Side of Enterprise**. New York: McGraw-Hill, 1960.
60. Stogdill, R. M., and Coons, A. E., 1957.
61. Maslow, A. H. **Motivation and Personality**. New York: Harper & Row, 1954.

UNIT 2   THE LEADER

One of the concerns of every leader is the relationship between leader and follower; how to cause others to be motivated to perform desired goals or outcomes. In this unit we will concentrate on the core of our model, the leader's relationship to those being led. Since leadership involves human interaction, it is well to focus on some common human characteristics shared by leaders and those being led. Sensitivity to these commonalities makes the leader more aware that accomplishment of work goals depends on the human resource, people. The leader needs to be concerned with the wants and desires of people, as these wants and desires affect the level of production attained.

Maslow believes that people want to maintain their dignity and to have a feeling of self-esteem. He wrote that one seeks [1]:

To be a prime mover
Self-determination
To have control over one's own fate
To determine one's movements
To be able to plan and carry out and to succeed
To expect success
To like responsibility or at any rate to assume it willingly, especially for one's self
To be active rather than passive
To be a person rather than a thing
To experience one's self as the maker of one's own decisions
Autonomy
Initiative
Self-starting
To have others acknowledge one's capabilities fairly

Reprinted with permission. Abraham Maslow, *Eupsychian Management*, (Homewood, Ill.: Richard D. Irwin, 1965), p. 45. ©1965 by Richard D. Irwin, Inc.

Maslow wrote about behaviors exhibited by people who are dominated or not respected. He stated that people react in certain ways to maintain their dignity, which he expressed as shown in Exhibit 2-1 [2].

Exhibit 2-1.   Maslow's Chart of Followers' Dislikes and Behaviors

Human beings avoid	To be a nothing (rather than a something)	A ludicrous figure regulated by others (like an object, to be treated like a physical object rather than like a person; to be rubricized, like an example rather than as unique)
Being Manipulated Dominated Pushed around Determined by others Misunderstood	Unappreciated Not respected Not feared Not taken seriously Laughed at	Given orders Forced Screwed (used, exploited, raped) Controlled Helpless Compliant Deferent An interchangeable man

Reprinted with permission. Abraham Maslow, *Eupsychian Management*, (Homewood, Ill.: Richard D. Irwin, 1965) p. 44. © 1965 by Richard D. Irwin, Inc.

A leader's philosophy of life is a key ingredient in how that leader relates to followers. No one likes to be dominated or misunderstood or any of the other "dislikes" that Maslow included in his chart. As a leader, you can begin analyzing your own philosophy by questioning how you feel about yourself. How do you respond to those who are your leaders? How does your relationship with your leader(s) affect your relationship with those you lead?

Again quoting from Maslow:

And now I would ask the question, "How can any human being help but be insulted by being treated as an interchangeable part, as simply a cog in a machine, as no more than an appurtenance to an assembly line (an appurtenance less good than a good machine)? There is no other human, reasonable, intelligible way to respond to this kind of profound cutting off of half of one's growth possibilities than by getting angry or resentful or struggling to get out of the situation. [3]

Reprinted with permission. Abraham Maslow, *Eupsychian Management*, (Homewood, Ill.: Richard D. Irwin, 1965), p. 47. © 1965 by Richard D. Irwin, Inc.

The first selection in this unit deals with maintenance of dignity and "dislikes" or effects of loss of dignity that can occur in workers from another viewpoint. Peter Drucker has written about differences in managing direct production workers and "knowledge workers." Drucker cited alienation of the knowledge worker as a problem in organizations that employ large numbers of educated persons. Nurses can be classified as knowledge workers since they have the benefit of post-secondary education and are paid for applying their knowledge in performing a public service. There is evidence that nurses do experience the social phenomenon of alienation in the workplace. Do leaders escape the phenomenon of alienation, or are they subject to the same feelings as are described in Drucker's article?

According to the definition of our model for leadership, the leader interacts with the workplace and often has a management role in that workplace. Drucker's article is written from a management perspective. Nurse-managers are knowledge workers, and the people they manage are often other knowledge workers. Both novice and experienced managers may find the points made in this article informative and useful. When reading it one may logically ask whether managers of knowledge workers must also be leaders.

Let us consider the feelings of novice managers. One of the conflicts experienced by these people is a feeling of intimidation when actively managing others with similar education or more experience or both. Does this feeling of intimidation stem from the manager's perception that he or she is not qualified to "lead" others with equal education? Does it stem from inexperience in applying the theories, concepts, and skills of management? Perhaps leadership is best developed through experiences in which one can test various leadership behaviors and inclinations in managing others. Perhaps some persons do not have the inclination to be leaders but can learn to be effective managers nonetheless.

Abraham Zaleznik contrasts managers and leaders in "Managers and Leaders: Are They Different?" This article is included for the purpose of giving you some content on which to base thoughtful consideration of management and leadership roles of a professional nurse. One problem in such reflection is the ambiguity in terminology used in common parlance about the two roles and also found in management literature. Zaleznik's comparison serves as a foil for explicating aspects of your professional role related to either leadership or management.

Zaleznik wrote of confrontation and of stripping away ambiguity—his article not only serves to help us define terms and explore concepts but also as a basis for confronting ourselves. What are our talents? What are our goals? How do we want to relate to other people? How do we want to relate to the organization that employs us? How do we want to relate to our profession? A leader can experience confrontation in many ways. One can confront other people, barriers of many different types such as regulations, policies or rules, and inanimate objects. The outcomes of confrontation depend on the relative strengths of the "objects" involved and the forces of the confrontation.

Let us posit that the leader's strengths are internal to the person and include personality, aptitudes, knowledge, self-awareness, and other personal attributes. Motivation, commitment, and energy are some of the leader's forces. If this concept of leader's strength and force is plausible, the leader must confront self to analyze the nature of his or her strengths and forces before effectively confronting others from a leadership position. In our introductory model, the core or leader strengths influence the impact that the leader will have when interacting with the environmental components.

The next article in this unit, Norman Hill's "Self-Esteem, The Key To Effective Leadership" relates leadership styles to the leader's own self-esteem. The theme is again that leaders' behaviors influence others. There is a dichotomy between this article and Zaleznik's that stems from ambiguous use of terminology. Hill's article defines leadership as working with people and promoting their growth, while Zaleznik's leaves the reader with the question of whether the "intense motivation" of leaders represents wasted energy or high performance. Hill's inferences of "leadership behaviors" more closely match those termed "management behaviors" by Zaleznik. In nursing education, we tend to teach students to become leaders in the terms that Hill elaborates rather than in Zaleznik's terms.

Zaleznik wrote that managers are developed through socialization whereas leaders are developed through personal mastery. This statement should cause us to question how nursing students develop leadership skills. Many aspects of nursing education emphasize socialization into the professional role through both educational content and group-oriented processes such as large classes and enrollment in nursing courses with learning activities defined for students within the time frame of an academic term. Do these circumscribed learning experiences develop leaders through either personal mastery or socialization processes? By the same token, the organization of nurses in staffing patterns such as functional and team nursing emphasize social relationships in the workplace. Do these staffing patterns promote the development of management skills or of leadership? Does the primary nursing model shift the emphasis from socialization in a group role to mastery of self and thus does it promote leadership development? These are all very pertinent questions for a profession that is concerned with continuing to develop leaders. In this regard let us question use of the terms leader and manager.

Attention must be paid to the development of leaders not only in educational programs but also in the workplace. James MacGregor Burns wrote that:

> *Qualities of leadership emerge out of . . . initiative, selective, and role taking or empathetic processes. As persons gain experience, knowledge and understanding, imitation, intentionality, and capacity for higher moral judgment, and as they grow more skillful in accommodation and role-taking, they gain in the capacity for leadership that draws from understanding of others' needs, roles, and values and expresses fundamental principles and purposes. Distinctions emerge between leader and follower, for leaders must comprehend many roles and followers fewer: leaders must accommodate followers' wants and needs without sacrificing basic principle (otherwise they would not be leaders); they must mediate group conflict without becoming mere references or conciliators without purpose of their own; they must be "with" their followers but also above them. But the leader's main strength is the ability to operate close enough to the followers to draw them up to the leader's level of moral development. [4]*

From this quotation, one can assume that educational preparation for leadership within the context of a term or even an entire nursing program is not adequate to stimulate the emergence of leaders. Close relationships with followers, and, we should add, all of the relationships involved in the work of patient care in an organization or other structure of employment, occur over time. Moral development in the context of a profession is initiated in an educational program, but we can posit that it is not internalized until one has tested oneself in the long-term practice of the profession in the workplace. If one is to maintain a "purpose of his own," attaining the ideals of patient care learned in school occurs through using strategies developed in relation to the issues in the practice setting. The strategies or pathways to achieving these ideals are the worker's contribution cited by Drucker that, when met, more closely align practice with the ideal design.

You may prefer to label Zaleznik's "leader" a superleader and his manager a leader, as described in the introduction to this anthology. At this point, you may be feeling that the precise definitions of management and leadership are not that necessary for resolving practical difficulties in the workplace such as presented by Drucker—how to evaluate the productivity of knowledge workers and how to prevent their alienation.

A more precise definition of leadership, however, may be relevant to defining leadership within the professional nursing organizations. Zaleznik's leaders (persons who stimulate intensive individual motivation in others and who are risk-takers) may be the type of person needed to carry out the future-oriented activities of the professional nursing organizations. Should leaders in professional nursing organizations be different from leaders in the workplace?

Sensitivity to the feelings of others is an underlying theme in this section. The last article, written by William C. Parrish, illustrates the point that the way leaders perceive themselves and others in-fluences their styles of leadership. Parrish dealt with the issue raised by Drucker that people are valuable and expensive resources, and that there is a great monetary investment in each knowledge worker. Parrish elaborated this theme by relating the effects of management and leadership to levels of productivity, retention of personnel, to use of time, energy, and organizational resources—all matters which have implications for the cost of nursing care. People determine and hence control the productivity of labor-intensive organizations such as health care agencies. The costs of leadership styles then are not only the emotional costs for people involved, but also the real dollar costs for an organization.

It should be noted that Parrish stated that "leaders are managers." Was he implying that leadership is a function of management closely aligned with human relations skills? Or is one characteristic of the leader the ability to manage? How does this contrast with Zaleznik's use of the term management as dealing with substantive resources? Are people substantive resources? Consider the following quote from Maslow. It provides food for thoughtful leaders—or managers?—and brings us back to the statements about what people want and need:

psychodynamic understanding of self-esteem and of dignity would make a great dif-ference in the industrial situation because the feelings of dignity, of respect and of self-respect are so easy to give! It costs little or nothing, it's a matter of an attitude, a deep-lying sympathy and understanding which can express itself almost auto-matically in various ways that can be quite satisfying, since they save the dignity of the person. [5]

MANAGING THE KNOWLEDGE WORKER

By Peter F. Drucker

TWO NEEDS

We do not know how to measure either the productivity or the satisfaction of the knowledge worker. But we do know quite a bit about improving both. Indeed the two needs: the need of business and the economy for productive knowledge workers and the need of the knowledge worker for achievement, while distinctly separate, are by and large satisfied by the same approaches to managing the knowledge worker.

1. We know first that the key to both the productivity of the knowledge worker and his achievement is to demand responsibility from him or her. All knowledge workers, from the lowliest and youngest to the company's chief executive officer, should be asked at least once a year: "What do you **contribute** that justifies your being on the payroll? What should this company, this hospital, this government agency, this university, hold you accountable for, by way of contributions and results? Do you know what your goals and objectives are? And what do you plan to do to attain them?"

Direction of the knowledge worker toward contribution—rather than toward effort alone—is the first job of anyone who manages knowledge workers. It is rarely even attempted. Often the engineering department only finds out, after it has finished the design, that the product on which it has been working so hard has no future in the marketplace.

2. But at the same time, the knowledge worker must be able to appraise his contribution. It is commonly said that research is "intangible" and incapable even of being appraised. But this is simply untrue.

Wherever a research department truly performs (an exception, alas, rather than the rule), the members sit down with each other and with management once or twice a year and think through two questions: "What have we contributed in the last two or three years that really made a difference to this company?" and "What should we be trying to contribute the next two or three years so as to make a difference?"

The contributions may indeed not always be measurable. How to judge them may be controversial. What, for instance, is a greater "contribution": a new biochemical discovery that after five more years of very hard work may lead to the development of a new class of medicinal compounds with superior properties; or the development of a sugar-coated aspirin without great "scientific value" that will improve the effec-

75

tiveness of pediatric medicine by making the aspirin more palatable for children, while also immediately increasing the company's sales and profits?

In fact, unless knowledge workers are made to review, appraise and judge, they will not direct themselves toward contribution. And they will also feel dissatisfied, nonachieving and altogether "alienated."

3. Perhaps the most important rule—and the one to which few managements pay much attention—is to enable the knowledge workers to do what they are being paid for. Not to be able to do what one is being paid for infallibly quenches whatever motivation there is. Yet salesmen, who are being paid for selling and know it, cannot sell because of the time demands of the paperwork imposed on them by management. And in research lab after research lab, highly paid and competent scientists are not allowed to do their work, but are instead forced to attend endless meetings to which they cannot contribute and from which they get nothing.

The manager may know the rule. But rarely does he know what he or the company does that impedes knowledge workers and gets in the way of their doing what they are being paid for. There is only one way to find out: Ask the individual knowledge worker (and the knowledge-work team he belongs to): "What do I, as your manager, and what do we in the company's management altogether, do that helps you in doing what you are being paid for?" "What do we do that hampers you?" "Specifically, do we give you the time to do what you are being paid for, the information you need to do it, the tools for the job?"

4. Knowledge is a high-grade resource. And knowledge workers are expensive. Their placement is therefore a key to their productivity. The first rule is that opportunities have to be staffed with people capable of running with them and of turning them into results. To make knowledge workers pro-

ductive requires constant attention to what management consulting firms and law firms call "assignment control." One has to know where the people are who are capable of producing results in knowledge work—precisely because results are so very hard to measure.

Effective management of the knowledge worker requires a regular, periodic inventory and ranking of the major opportunities. And then one asks: "Who are the performing people available to us, whether they are researchers or accountants, salesmen or managers, manufacturing engineers or economic analysts? And what are these people assigned to? Are they where the results are? Or are their assignments such that they could not produce real results, no matter how well they perform?"

Unless this is being done, people will be assigned by the demands of the organization—that is by the number of transactions rather than by their importance and their potential of contribution. In no time they will be misassigned. They will be where they cannot be productive, no matter how well motivated, how highly qualified, how dedicated they are.

One also has to make sure that knowledge workers are placed where their strengths can be productive. There are no universal geniuses, least of all in knowledge work, which tends to be highly specialized. What can this particular knowledge worker do? What is he doing well? And where, therefore, does he truly belong to get the greatest results from his strengths?

Most businesses and other organizations as well spend a great deal of time and money on the original employment of people who, it is hoped, will turn into knowledge workers. But at that stage one knows very little about the future employee—beyond the grades he got in school, which have little correlation with future performance capacity. The true personnel management job, in respect to knowledge workers, begins later, when one can place the worker where his strengths can be productive because one knows what he or she can do.

SKILLS AND ABILITY

Manual strength is additive. Two oxen will pull almost twice the load one ox can pull. Skill is capable of subdivision. Three men, each of whom has learned one aspect of a skill, e.g., glueing the legs to a table, can turn out far more work of equal skill than one man skilled in all aspects of carpentry. But in knowledge work two mediocre people do not turn out more than one man capable of performance, let alone twice as much. They tend to get in each other's way, and to turn out much less than one capable person. In knowledge work, above all, one therefore has to staff from strength. And this means constant attention to placing the knowledge worker where what he can do will produce results and make a contribution.

Knowledge is perhaps the most expensive of all resources. Knowledge workers are far more expensive than even their salaries indicate. Each of them also represents a very sizeable capital investment—in schooling and in the apprentice years during which the worker learns rather than contributes (such as the five years which every chief engineer knows will be needed before the young graduate can truly be expected to earn his salary). Every young engineer, every young accountant, every young market researcher represents a "social capital investment" of something like $100,000 to $150,000 before he starts repaying society and his employer through his contributions. No other resource we have is equally "capital intensive" and "labor intensive." And only management can turn the knowledge worker into a productive resource.

But also, no one expects to achieve, to produce, to contribute quite as much as the knowledge worker does. No one, in other words, is more likely to be "alienated" if not allowed to achieve.

Not to manage a knowledge worker for productivity therefore creates both the economic stress of inflationary pressures and the highly contagious social disease of distemper. We can indeed measure neither the productivity nor the satisfaction of the knowledge worker. But we know how to enrich both.

MANAGERS AND LEADERS: ARE THEY DIFFERENT?

By Abraham Zaleznik

Reprinted from *Harvard Business Review*, May–June 1977, Copyright © 1977 by the President and Fellows of Harvard College; all rights reserved.

Most societies, and that includes business organizations, are caught between two conflicting needs: one, for managers to maintain the balance of operations, and one for leaders to create new approaches and imagine new areas to explore. One might well ask why there is a conflict. Cannot both managers and leaders exist in the same society, or even better, cannot one person be both a manager and a leader?

What is the ideal way to develop leadership? Every society provides its own answer to this question, and each, in groping for answers, defines its deepest concerns about the purposes, distributions, and uses of power. Business has contributed its answer to the leadership question by evolving a new breed called the manager. Simultaneously, business has established a new power ethic that favors collective over individual leadership, the cult of the group over that of personality. While ensuring the competence, control, and the balance of power relations among groups with the potential for rivalry, managerial leadership unfortunately does not necessarily ensure imagination, creativity, or ethical behavior in guiding the destinies of corporate enterprises.

Leadership inevitably requires using power to influence the thoughts and actions of other people. Power in the hands of an individual entails human risks: first, the risk of equating power with the ability to get immediate results; second, the risk of ignoring the many different ways people can legitimately accumulate power; and third, the risk of losing self-control in the desire for power. The need to hedge these risks accounts in part for the development of collective leadership and the managerial ethic. Consequently, an inherent conservatism dominates the culture of large organizations. In **The Second American Revolution**, John D. Rockefeller, 3rd describes the conservatism of organizations:

An organization is a system with a logic of its own and all the weight of tradition and inertia. The deck is stacked in favor of the tried and proven way of doing things and against the taking of risks and striking out in new directions. [6]

Out of this conservatism and inertia organizations provide succession to power through the development of managers rather than individual leaders. And the irony of the managerial ethic is that it fosters a bureaucratic culture in business, supposedly the last bastion protecting us from the encroachments and controls of bureaucracy in government and education. Perhaps the risks associated with power in the hands of an individual may be necessary ones for business to take if organizations are to break free of their inertia and bureaucratic conservatism.

MANAGER VS. LEADER PERSONALITY

Theodore Levitt has described the essential features of a managerial culture with its emphasis on rationality and control:

Management consists of the rational assessment of a situation and the systematic selection of goals and purposes (what is to be done?); the systematic development of strategies to achieve these goals; the marshalling of the required resources; the rational design, organization, direction, and control of the activities required to attain the selected purposes; and, finally, the motivating and rewarding of people to do the work. [7]

In other words, whether his or her energies are directed toward goals, resources, organization structures, or people, a manager is a problem-solver. The manager asks himself, "What problems have to be solved, and what are the best ways to achieve results so that people will continue to contribute to this organization?" In this conception, leadership is a practical effort to direct affairs; and to fulfill his task, a manager requires that many people operate at different levels of status and responsibility. Our democratic society is, in fact, unique in having solved the problem of providing well-trained managers for business. The same solution stands ready to be applied to government, education, health care, and other institutions. It takes neither genius nor heroism to be a manager, but rather persistence, tough-mindedness, hard work, intelligence, analytical ability and, perhaps most important, tolerance and good will.

Another conception, however, attaches almost mystical beliefs to what leadership is and assumes that only great people are worthy of the drama of power and politics. Here, leadership is a psychodrama in which, as a precondition for control of a political structure, a lonely person must gain control of himself or herself. Such an expectation of leadership contrasts sharply with the mundane, practical, and yet important conception that leadership is really managing work that other people do.

Two questions come to mind. Is this mystique of leadership merely a holdover from our collective childhood of dependency and our longing for good and heroic parents? Or, is there a basic truth lurking behind the need for leaders that no matter how competent managers are, their leadership stagnates because of their limitations in visualizing purposes and generating value in work? Without this imaginative capacity and the ability to communicate, managers, driven by their narrow purposes, perpetuate group conflicts instead of reforming them into broader desires and goals.

If indeed problems demand greatness, then, judging by past performance, the selection and development of leaders leave a great deal to chance. There are no known ways to train "great" leaders. Furthermore, beyond what we leave to chance, there is a deeper issue in the relation between the need for competent managers and the longing for great leaders.

What it takes to ensure the supply of people who will assume practical responsibility may inhibit the development of great leaders. Conversely, the presence of great leaders may undermine the development of managers who become very anxious in the relative disorder that leaders seem to generate. The antagonism in aim (to have many competent managers as well as great leaders) often remains obscure in stable and well-developed societies. But the antagonism surfaces during periods of stress and change, as it did in the Western countries during both the Great Depression and World War II. The tension also appears in the struggle for power between theorists and professional managers in revolutionary societies.

It is easy enough to dismiss the dilemma I pose (of training managers while we may need new leaders, or leaders at the expense of managers) by saying that the need is for people who can be **both** managers and leaders. The truth of the matter as I see it, however, is that just as a managerial culture is different from the entrepreneurial culture that develops when leaders appear in organizations, managers and leaders are very different kinds of people. They differ in motivation, personal history, and in how they think and act.

A technologically oriented and economically successful society tends to depreciate the need for great leaders. Such societies hold a deep and abiding faith in rational methods of solving problems, including problems of value, economics, and justice. Once rational methods of solving problems are broken down into elements, organized, and taught as skills, then society's faith in technique over personal qualities in leadership remains the guiding conception for a democratic society contemplating its leadership requirements. But there are times when tinkering and trial and error prove inadequate to the emerging problems of selecting goals, allocating resources, and distributing wealth and opportunity. During such times, the democratic society needs to find leaders who use themselves as the instruments of learning and acting, instead of managers who use their accumulation of collective experience to get where they are going.

Managers and leaders differ fundamentally in their world views. The dimensions for assessing these differences include managers' and leaders' orientations toward their goals, their work, their human relations, and their selves.

Attitudes toward Goals

Managers tend to adopt impersonal, if not passive, attitudes toward goals. Managerial goals arise out of necessities rather than desires, and, therefore, are deeply embedded in the history and culture of the organization.

Frederic G. Donner, chairman and chief executive officer of General Motors from 1958 to 1967, expressed this impersonal and passive attitude toward goals in defining GM's position on product development:

To meet the challenge of the marketplace, we must recognize changes in customer needs and desires far enough ahead to have the right products in the right places at the right time and in the right quantity.

We must balance trends in preference against the many compromises that are necessary to make a final product that is both reliable and good looking, that performs well and that sells at a competitive price in the necessary volume. We must design, not just the cars we would like to build, but more importantly, the cars that our customers want to buy.

Nowhere in this formulation of how a product comes into being is there a notion that consumer tastes and preferences arise in part as a result of what manufacturers do.

The nurse-manager meets challenges in providing patient care services mandated by the patient census—covering and making do with scarce resources. This person determines goals according to the number of patients and their needs for basic care, keeping the lid on situations rather than determining goals of quality care or types of care he or she might desire. To paraphrase the preceding quote from the General Motors executive, such a nurse-manager might argue:

We must balance trends in preference against the many compromises that are necessary to provide care that is efficacious and of high quality, and that patients given a choice, would select in a competitive health care industry. We must design, not just the care we would like to give, but more importantly the care that our patients want to buy.

And we can paraphrase Zaleznik's analysis of this way of thinking, to point out that nowhere in this formulation of how care can be given is there a notion that patients' tastes and preferences arise in part as a result of what nurses do.

In reality, through product (or health care) design, advertising, and promotion, consumers learn to like what they then say they need. Few would argue that people who enjoy taking snapshots **need** a camera that also develops pictures. But in response to novelty, convenience, a shorter interval between acting (taking the snap) and gaining pleasure (seeing the shot), the Polaroid camera succeeded in the marketplace. But it is inconceivable that Edwin Land responded to impressions of consumer need. Instead, he translated a technology (polarization of light) into a product, which proliferated and stimulated consumers' desires.

The example of Polaroid and Land suggests how leaders think about goals. They are active instead of reactive, shaping ideas instead of responding to them. Leaders adopt a personal and active attitude toward goals. The influence a leader exerts in altering moods, evoking images and expectations, and in establishing specific desires and objectives determines the direction a business takes. The net result of this influence is to change the way people think about what is desirable, possible, and necessary.

Conceptions of Work

What do managers and leaders do? What is the nature of their respective work?

Leaders and managers differ in their conceptions. Managers tend to view work as an enabling process involving some combina-tion of people and ideas interacting to establish strategies and make decisions. Managers help the process along by a range of skills, including calculating the interests in opposition, staging and timing the surfacing of controversial issues, and reducing tensions. In this enabling process, managers appear flexible in the use of tactics: they negotiate and bargain, on the one hand, and use rewards and punishments, and other forms of coercion, on the other. Machiavelli wrote for managers and not necessarily for leaders.

In order to get people to accept solutions to problems, managers need to coordinate and balance continually. Interestingly enough, this managerial work has much in common with what diplomats and mediators do. The manager aims at shifting balances of power toward solutions acceptable as a compromise among conflicting values.

What about leaders: what do they do? Where managers act to limit choices, leaders work in the opposite direction, to develop fresh approaches to long-standing problems and to open issues for new options. Stanley and Inge Hoffmann, the political scientists, liken the leader's work to that of the artist. But unlike most artists, the leader himself is an integral part of the aesthetic product. One cannot look at a leader's art without looking at the artist. On Charles de Gaulle as a political artist, they wrote: "And each of his major political acts, however tortuous the means or the details, has been whole, indivisible and unmistakably his own, like an artistic act" [8].

The closest one can get to a product apart from the artist is the ideas that occupy, indeed at times obsess, the leader's mental life. To be effective, however, the leader needs to project his ideas into images that excite people, and only then develop choices that give the projected images substance. Consequently, leaders create excitement in work.

Leaders working from high-risk positions indeed often are temperamentally disposed to seek out risk and danger, especially where opportunity and reward appear high. From my observations, why one individual seeks risks while another approaches problems conservatively depends more on his or her personality and less on conscious choice. For some, especially those who become managers, the instinct for survival dominates their need for risk, and their ability to tolerate mundane, practical work assists their survival. The same cannot be said for leaders, who sometimes react to mundane work as to an affliction.

Relations with Others

Managers prefer to work with people; they avoid solitary activity because it makes them anxious. Several years ago, I directed studies on the psychological aspects of career. The need to seek out others with whom to work and collaborate seemed to stand out as important characteristics of managers. When asked, for example, to write imaginative stories in response to a picture showing a single figure (a boy contemplating a violin, or a man silhouetted in a state of reflection), managers populated their stories with people. The following is an example of a manager's imaginative story about the young boy contemplating a violin:

Mom and Dad insisted that junior take music lessons so that someday he can become a concert musician. His instrument was ordered and had just arrived. Junior is weighing the alternatives of playing football with the other kids or playing with the squeak box. He can't understand how his parents could think a violin is better than a touchdown.

After four months of practicing the violin, junior has had more than enough, Daddy is going out of his mind, and Mommy is willing to give in reluctantly to the men's wishes. Football season is now over but a good third baseman will take the field next spring. [9]

This story illustrates two themes that clarify managerial attitudes toward human relations. The first, as I have suggested, is to seek out activity with other people (i.e., the football team), and the second is to maintain a low level of emotional involvement in these relationships. The low emotional involvement appears in the writer's use of conventional metaphors, even clichés, and in the depiction of the ready transformation of potential conflict into harmonious decisions. In this case, Junior, Mommy, and Daddy agree to give up the violin for manly sports.

These two themes may seem paradoxical, but their coexistence supports what a manager does, including reconciling differences, seeking compromises, and establishing a balance of power. A further idea demonstrated by how the manager wrote the story is that managers may lack empathy, or the capacity to sense intuitively the thoughts and feelings of others. To illustrate attempts to be empathic, here is another story written to the same stimulus picture by someone considered by his peers to be a leader.

This little boy has the appearance of being a sincere artist, one who is deeply affected by the violin, and has an intense desire to master the instrument.

He seems to have just completed his normal practice session and appears to be somewhat crestfallen at his inability to produce the sounds which he is sure lie within the violin.

He appears to be in the process of making a vow to himself to expend the necessary time and effort to play this instrument until he satisfies himself that he is able to bring forth the qualities of music which he feels within himself.

With this type of determination and carry through, this boy became one of the great violinists of his day. [10]

Empathy is not simply a matter of paying attention to other people. It is also the capacity to take in emotional signals and to make them mean something in a relationship with an individual. People who describe another person as "deeply affected" with "intense desire," as capable of feeling "crestfallen" and as one who can "vow to himself," would seem to have an inner perceptiveness that they can use in their relationships with others.

Managers relate to people according to the role they play in a sequence of events or in a decision-making **process**, while leaders, who are concerned with ideas, relate in more intuitive and empathetic ways. The manager's orientation to people, as actors in a sequence of events, deflects his or her attention away from the substance of people's concerns and toward their roles in a process. The distinction is simply between a manager's attention to **how** things get done and a leader's to **what** the events and decisions mean to participants.

In recent years, managers have taken over from game theory the notion that decision-making events can be one of two types: the win-lose situation (or zero-sum game) or the win-win situation in which everybody in the action comes out ahead. As part of the process of reconciling differences among people and maintaining balances of power, managers strive to convert win-lose into win-win situations.

As an illustration, take the decision of how to allocate capital resources among operating divisions in a large, decentralized organization. On the face of it, the dollars available for distribution are limited at any given time. Presumably, therefore, the more one division gets, the less is available for other divisions.

Managers tend to view this situation (as it affects human relations) as a conversion issue: how to make what seems like a win-lose problem into a win-win problem. Several solutions to this situation come to mind. First, the manager focuses others' attention on procedure and not on substance. Here the actors become engrossed in the bigger problem of **how** to make decisions, not **what** decisions to make. Once committed to the bigger problem, the actors have to support the outcome since they were involved in formulating decision rules. Because the actors believe in the rules they formulated, they will accept present losses in the expectation that next time they will win.

Second, the manager communicates to his subordinates indirectly, using "signals" instead of "messages." A signal has a number of possible implicit positions in it while a message clearly states a position. Signals are inconclusive and subject to reinterpretation should people become upset and angry, while messages involve the direct consequence that some people will indeed not like what they hear. The nature of messages heightens emotional response, and, as I have indicated, emotionally makes managers anxious. With signals, the question of who wins and who loses often becomes obscured.

Third, the manager plays for time. Managers seem to recognize that with the passage of time and the delay of major decisions, compromises emerge that take the sting out of win-lose situations; and the original "game" will be superseded by additional ones. Therefore, compromises may mean that one wins and loses simultaneously, depending on which of the games one evaluates.

There are undoubtedly many other tactical moves managers use to change human situations from win-lose to win-win. But the point to be made is that such tactics focus on the decision-making process itself and interest managers rather than leaders. The interest in tactics involves costs as well as benefits, including making organizations fatter in bureaucratic and political intrigue and leaner in direct, hard activity and warm human relationships. Consequently, one often hears subordinates characterize managers as inscrutable, detached, and manipulative. These adjectives arise from the subordinates' perception that they are linked together in a process whose purpose, beyond simply making decisions, is to maintain a controlled as well as rational and equitable structure. These adjectives suggest that managers need order in the face of the potential chaos that many fear in human relationships.

In contrast, one often hears leaders referred to in adjectives rich in emotional content. Leaders attract strong feelings of identity and difference, or of love and hate. Human relations in leader-dominated structures often appear turbulent, intense, and at times even disorganized. Such an atmosphere intensifies individual motivation and often produces unanticipated outcomes. Does this intense motivation lead to innovation and high performance, or does it represent wasted energy?

Senses of Self

In **The Varieties of Religious Experience,** William James describes two basic personality types, "once-born" and "twice-born" [11]. People of the former personality type are those for whom adjustments to life have been straightforward and whose lives have been more or less a peaceful flow from the moment of their births. The twice-borns, on the other hand, have not had an easy time of it. Their lives are marked by a continual struggle to attain some sense of order. Unlike the once-borns they cannot take things for granted. According to James, these personalities have equally different world views. For a once-born personality, the sense of self, as a guide to conduct and attitude, derives from a feeling of being at home and in harmony with one's environment. For a twice-born, the sense of self derives from a feeling of profound separateness.

A sense of belonging or of being separate has a practical significance for the kinds of investments managers and leaders make in their careers. Managers see themselves as conservators and regulators of an existing order of affairs with which they personally identify and from which they gain rewards. Perpetuating and strengthening existing institutions enhances a manager's sense of self-worth: he or she is performing in a role that harmonizes with the ideals of duty and responsibility. William James had this harmony in mind—this sense of self as flowing easily to and from the outer world—in defining a once-born personality. If one feels oneself as a member of institutions, contributing to their well-being, then one fulfills a mission in life and feels rewarded for having measured up to ideals. This reward transcends material gains and answers the more fundamental desire for personal integrity which is achieved by identifying with existing institutions.

Leaders tend to be twice-born personalities, people who feel separate from their environment, including other people. They may work in organizations, but they never belong to them. Their sense of who they are does not depend upon memberships, work roles, or other social indicators of identity. What seems to follow from this idea about separateness is some theoretical basis for explaining why certain individuals search out opportunities for change. The methods to bring about change may be technological, political, or ideological, but the object is the same: to profoundly alter human, economic, and political relationships.

Sociologists refer to the preparation individuals undergo to perform in roles as the socialization process. Where individuals experience themselves as an integral part of the social structure (their self-esteem gains strength through participation and conformity), social standards exert powerful effects in maintaining the individual's personal sense of continuity, even beyond the early years in the family. The line of development from the family to schools, then to career is cumulative and reinforcing. When the line of development is not reinforcing because of significant disruptions in relationships or other problems experienced in the family or other social institutions, the individual turns inward and struggles to establish self-esteem, identity, and order. Here the psychological dynamics center on the experience with loss and the efforts at recovery.

In considering the development of leadership, we have to examine two different courses of life history: 1) development through socialization, which prepares the individual to guide institutions and to maintain the existing balance of social relations; and 2) development through personal mastery, which impels an individual to struggle for psychological and social change. Society produces its managerial talent through the first line of development, while through the second leaders emerge.

DEVELOPMENT OF LEADERSHIP

The development of every person begins in the family. Each person experiences the traumas associated with separating from his or her parents, as well as the pain that follows such frustration. In the same vein, all individuals face the difficulties of achieving self-regulation and self-control. But for some, perhaps a majority, the fortunes of childhood provide adequate gratifications and sufficient opportunities to find substitutes for rewards no longer available. Such individuals, the "once-borns," make moderate identifications with parents and find a harmony between what they expect and what they are able to realize from life.

But suppose the pains of separation are amplified by a combination of parental demands and the individual's needs to the degree that a sense of isolation, of being special, and of wariness disrupts the bonds that attach children to parents and other authority figures? Under such conditions, and given a special aptitude, the origins of which remain mysterious, the person becomes deeply involved in his or her inner world at the expense of interest in the outer world. For such a person, self-esteem no longer depends solely upon positive attachments and real rewards. A form of self-reliance takes hold along with expectations of performance and achievement, and perhaps even the desire to do great works.

Such self-perceptions can come to nothing if the individual's talents are negligible. Even with strong talents, there are no guarantees that achievement will follow, let alone that the end result will be for good rather than evil. Other factors enter into development. For one thing, leaders are like artists and other gifted people, who often struggle with neuroses; their ability to function varies considerably even over the short run, and some potential leaders may lose the struggle altogether. Also, beyond early childhood, the patterns of development that affect managers and leaders involve the selective influence of particular people. Just as they appear flexible and evenly distributed in the types of talents available for development, managers form moderate and widely distributed attachments. Leaders, on the other hand, establish, and also break off, intensive one-to-one relationships.

It is a common observation that people with great talents are often only indifferent students. No one, for example, could have predicted Einstein's great achievements on the basis of his mediocre record in school. The reason for mediocrity is obviously not the absence of ability. It may result, instead, from self-absorption and the inability to pay attention to the ordinary tasks at hand. The only sure way an individual can interrupt reverielike preoccupation and self-absorption is to form a deep attachment to a great teacher or other benevolent person who understands and has the ability to communicate with the gifted individual.

Whether gifted individuals find what they need in one-to-one relationships depends on the availability of sensitive and intuitive mentors who have a vocation in cultivating talent. Fortunately, when the generations do meet and the self-selections occur, we learn more about how to develop leaders and how talented people of different generations influence each other.

While apparently destined for a mediocre career, people who form important one-to-one relationships are able to accelerate and intensify their development through an apprenticeship. The background for such apprenticeships, or the psychological readiness of an individual to benefit from an intensive relationship, depends upon some experience in life that forces the individual to turn inward.

Psychological biographies of gifted people repeatedly demonstrate the important part a mentor plays in developing an individual. Andrew Carnegie owed much to his senior, Thomas A. Scott. As head of the Western Division of the Pennsylvania Railroad, Scott recognized talent and the desire to learn in the young telegrapher assigned to him. By giving Carnegie increasing responsibility and by providing him with the opportunity to learn through close personal observation, Scott added to Carnegie's self-confidence and sense of achievement. Because of his own personal strength and achievement, Scott did not fear Carnegie's aggressiveness. Rather, he gave it full play in encouraging Carnegie's initiative.

Mentors take risks with people. They bet initially on talent they perceive in younger people. Mentors also risk emotional involvement in working closely with their juniors. The risks do not always pay off, but the willingness to take them appears crucial in developing leaders.

CAN ORGANIZATIONS DEVELOP LEADERS?

The examples I have given of how leaders develop suggest the importance of personal influence and the one-to-one relationship. For organizations to encourage consciously the development of leaders as compared with managers would mean developing one-to-one relationships between junior and senior executives and, more important, fostering a culture of individualism and possibly elitism. The elitism arises out of the desire to identify talent and other qualities suggestive of the ability to lead and not simply to manage.

A myth about how people learn and develop that seems to have taken hold in the American culture also dominates thinking in business. The myth is that people learn best from their peers. Supposedly, the threat of evaluation and even humiliation recedes in peer relations because of the tendency for mutual identification and the social restraints on authoritarian behavior among equals. Peer training in organizations occurs in various forms. The use, for example, of task forces made up of peers from several interested occupational groups (sales, production, research, and finance) supposedly removes the restraints of authority on the individual's willingess to assert and exchange ideas. As a result, so the theory goes, people interact more freely, listen more objectively to criticism and other points of view and, finally, learn from this healthy interchange.

Another application of peer training exists in some large corporations, such as Philips, N.V. in Holland, where organization structure is built on the principle of joint responsibility of two peers, one representing the commercial end of the business and the other the technical. Formally, both hold equal responsibility for geographic operations or product groups, as the case may be. As a practical matter, it may turn out that one or the other of the peers dominates the management. Nevertheless, the main interaction is between two or more equals.

The principal question I would raise about such arrangements is whether they perpetuate the managerial orientation, and preclude the formation of one-to-one relationships between senior people and potential leaders.

Aware of the possible stifling effects of peer relationships on aggressiveness and individual initiative, another company, much smaller then Philips, utilizes joint responsibility of peers for operating units, with one important difference. The chief executive of this company encourages competition and rivalry among peers, ultimately appointing the one who comes out on top for increased responsibility. These hybrid arrangements produce some unintended consequences that can be disastrous. There is no easy way to limit rivalry. Instead, it permeates all levels of the operation and opens the way for the formation of cliques in an atmosphere of intrigue.

A large, integrated oil company has accepted the importance of developing leaders through the direct influence of senior on junior executives. One chairman and chief executive officer regularly selected one talented university graduate whom he appointed his special assistant, and with whom he would work closely for a year. At the end of the year, the junior executive would become available for assignment to one of the operating divisions, where he would be assigned to a responsible post rather than a training position. The mentor relationship had acquainted the junior executive firsthand with the use of power, and with the important antidotes to the power disease called **hubris**—performance and integrity.

Working in one-to-one relationships, where there is a formal and recognized difference in the power of the actors, takes a great deal of tolerance for emotional interchange. This interchange, inevitable in close working arrangements, probably accounts for the reluctance of many executives to become involved in such relationships. **Fortune** carried an interesting story on the departure of a key executive, John W. Hanley, from the top management of

Procter & Gamble, for the chief executive officer position at Monsanto [12]. According to this account, the chief executive and chairman of P&G passed over Hanley for appointment to the presidency and named another executive vice president to this post instead.

The chairman evidently felt he could not work well with Hanley who, by his own acknowledgement, was aggressive, eager to experiment and change practices, and constantly challenged his superior. A chief executive officer naturally has the right to select people with whom he feels congenial. But I wonder whether a greater capacity on the part of senior officers to tolerate the competitive impulses and behavior of their subordinates might not be healthy for corporations. At least a greater tolerance for interchange would not favor the managerial team player at the expense of the individual who might become a leader.

I am constantly surprised at the frequency with which chief executives feel threatened by open challenges to their ideas, as though the source of their authority, rather than their specific ideas, were at issue. In one case a chief executive officer, who was troubled by the aggressiveness and sometimes outright rudeness of one of his talented vice presidents, used various indirect methods such as group meetings and hints from outside directors to avoid dealing with his subordinate. I advised the executive to deal head-on with what irritated him. I suggested that by direct, face-to-face confrontation, both he and his subordinate would learn to validate the distinction between the authority to be preserved and the issues to be debated.

To confront is also to tolerate aggressive interchange, and has the net effect of stripping away the veils of ambiguity and siganling so characteristic of managerial cultures, as well as encouraging the emotional relationship leaders need if they are to survive.

SELF-ESTEEM: THE KEY TO EFFECTIVE LEADERSHIP

By Norman Hill

Excerpted from *Administrative Management*, August 1976, copyright © 1976 by Geyer-McAllister Publications, Inc., New York.

Leadership is a process of influence. The process can be seen when people join together to accomplish some common objective through their collective efforts. Leadership refers to a person's ability to guide, modify, and direct the actions of others in such a way as to gain their cooperation in doing a job. It is the ability of a person to direct the problem-solving processes of others.

Three factors have been found which distinguish the most successful from the least successful leaders. These are integration toward goals, perseverance, and self-confidence. Apparently those who are the most successful recognize both their abilities and limitations, are reasonable in their aspirations and expectations, and are undaunted in pursuing them.

It seems that the reason those who possess a high degree of self-esteem are able to influence others is that their own sense of personal security is not violated in interpersonal exchanges. They feel neither threat nor insecurity because of their positive self-evaluation. In an organizational setting, such people are effective leaders because they exhibit the same confidence toward subordinates with which they regard themselves.

What leaders believe about themselves influences what they believe about subordinates. If they have confidence in their own ability, they will have high—but realistic—expectations of the people who report to them and help employees to satisfy what emerges as their mutual expectations. What leaders expect of them, and the subsequent way in which they treat the people who report to them, in turn largely determines their performance and development.

The influence of one person's expectations upon another's behavior has been demonstrated in organizational settings as well. David Berlew and Douglas Hall examined the career progress of managers employed by American Telephone and Telegraph Company. After observing 49 managers over a five-year period, they concluded that the relative success of managers, as indicated by promotions and estimates of each person's performance and potential, depended largely on their supervisors' expectations of them.

Several conclusions can be drawn about the influence leaders can exert through the expectations which they consistently maintain and demonstrate toward subordinates:

1. What leaders expect of their staffs affects their performance.

2. A unique characteristic of effective leaders is their ability to create high performance standards for the people who report to them to fulfill.

3. Ineffective leaders fail to develop the positive expectations and so subordinates accomplish less.

Those who occupy positions of authority in organizations are often more effective in communicating low expectations than they are in expressing high expectations. In fact, supervisors often communicate most when they think they are communicating least. What supervisors actually say matters less than how they behave. Expectations seem to be communicated most frequently by nonverbal cues such as the climate and norms a manager creates and perpetuates.

These unwritten rules, illustrated by the amount of attention and feedback given by a supervisor to subordinates, have the greatest amount of impact. Rewarding initiative, correcting mistakes, asking for input, sharing feelings, and being willing to change personal perceptions are some specific ways to communicate positive expectations.

To exert a meaningful influence, expectations must be more than the power of positive thinking. Harvard psychologist David McClelland has found that subordinates will not be influenced by a supervisor's expectations unless those expectations are considered reasonable and realistic. Goals that are too high or too low will have little impact on them. Influence seems greatest and motivation highest when subordinates feel that they have about a 50 percent probability—a 50/50 chance—of fulfilling their supervisors' explicit expectations.

Effective leaders seem to exhibit two common characteristics: confidence in their own ability and high expectations of others. The high expectations of effective leaders, moreover, are based primarily on how they feel about themselves. What people believe about themselves subtly influences what they believe about others, what they expect of them, and how they treat them. A leader who possesses a positive self-image will generate high performance standards from subordinates and will treat them with the confidence that these expectations and standards will be met. Expectations, then, become self-fulfilling if they appear reasonable and realistic to subordinates. So instead of saying "what you see is what you get," it could more appropriately be said that "what you expect is what you get."

IS FEAR A PART OF YOUR MANAGEMENT STYLE?

By William C. Parrish

Reprinted with permission from *Health Care Management Review*, Summer 1977. Published by Aspen Systems Corporation, Germantown, Maryland.

Many administrators, due to background, training, and their own personalities, adopt highly successful leadership patterns, while other patterns evolve less successfully. One leadership style—management by fear—is particularly noteworthy for its lack of success over the long run, yet it is seen repeatedly in varying degrees of severity in health care institutions.

Management by fear is the domination of subordinates through systematic application of formal authority, coercion, and oppressive controls. Management by fear uses threats and negative motivation to accomplish goals and objectives. Management by fear employs oral communications as a tool of domination, and subordinates often receive withering direct criticisms, along with generalized attacks on their competence, attitude, loyalty, and integrity.

To the administrator who uses it, this kind of leadership seems to get results because fear can be a powerful motivator over the short run. Whether a subordinate fears another tongue-lashing, a bad performance rating, a transfer to another job, or a loss of authority and responsibility, the result—a desire to avoid the outcome—is usually the same. This negative motivation pushes the subordinate toward goal-directed performance, often with zeal and dedication that must be satisfying to the leader, who becomes certain that he has found a surefire formula for success in his system of management by fear.

HUMAN RESOURCE COSTS

There are adverse effects of this leadership style. The human resource costs of a management-by-fear style of leadership can have many dimensions. One unaffordable dimension is that skilled professional and technical personnel are less inclined than ever to subject themselves to dehumanizing leadership. They may turn to unions as a buffer, or they simply pursue the alternative of least resistance: taking a usually readily available position with another hospital.

For those individuals who remain with the hospital, and there are, of course, many who cannot or will not leave, the other dimensions of the human resource costs of management by fear begin to take a toll on organizational effectiveness.

Management by fear resembles more benign and constructive forms of leadership much of the time. The leader makes decisions and interacts with others in a generally

91

normal fashion. The malignant aspects of management by fear may be triggered by seemingly routine minor events which the leader somehow perceives as a threat to his authority, a challenge to his dominance over everyone and everything in the organization, or a reduction of his power.

Consider, for example, the supervisor who receives a call from an irate family and in turn tells the newly appointed head nurse that she is an idiot to have let the family become irate. This response creates severe self-questioning and feelings of incompetence in a vulnerable person.

When employees are propelled into such unsettled emotional states, how much can they produce? What will be the quality of the health care they provide, or of the decisions they make?

The individual time lost can be substantial, but even more time is lost as individuals seek members of their peer groups to share experiences and feelings after a management-by-fear episode. In one hospital, a 15-minute coffee break for management and professional staff often stretched out to an hour as 10 or 12 staff members sought and gave emotional support.

The newly appointed head nurse might have sought solace from such a group.

SETTING THE STAGE

An administrator who practices management by fear is, of course, setting the stage for his subordinate managers to emulate him. The style of a senior leader is a key determinant in the style of leaders subordinate to him in the organization. In this way, the effects of a management-by-fear style can percolate downward through an entire organization.

In a hospital where management by fear is

utilized by top and middle layers of managers, the short-run results may look good as everyone is initially motivated to work twice as hard to avoid the consequences of not pleasing the boss, or missing a deadline, or making an honest mistake. Productivity may show a sharp increase, but, beneath the surface, factors of long-run significance will begin to emerge: positive attitudes toward the organization will slowly but inexorably change to negative attitudes. Hospital productivity may still look good at this point, but when attitudes have eroded enough, behavior itself begins to change adversely. Unproductive rather than productive kinds of behavior is the long-run performance outcome of the management-by-fear style.

Ultimately, management-by-fear leaders are harmful to their hospitals because of the huge human toll that they exact to obtain their short-run benefits. In a managment-by-fear environment, the subordinate has only four choices:

1. Withdraw from the painful environment by leaving the organization (very costly in recruiting, training, and start-up expenses)

2. Adapt by coasting (lower work standards, become apathetic, do the minimum required to get by, take no risks)

3. Adopt defensive mechanisms (fight the system or defend self-concepts; in either case, a normal result is to get quickly beaten down)

4. Deteriorate (anxiety reactions, situational maladjustment, ulcers, daydreaming)

Consider the choices that the novice head nurse might make—and consider the costs to the organization that might result from any one of those choices.

The health care field has many sensitive, effective leaders who can obtain maximum productivity from people while having maximum concern for the person, too. These leaders can be as tough as the management-by-fear leader in decision making, but one key difference is that the sensitive leader recognizes people as his most valuable asset and resource, whereas the management-by-fear leader has not or cannot come to grips with this critical fact of organizational life.

WHY?

Feelings toward Subordinates

What is it that causes some leaders to adopt a management-by-fear style while others, with perhaps the same training and experience, will adopt a more supportive, interpersonally successful style? One fundamental reason for this is the feelings that leaders have for their subordinates. These feelings in the leader are powerful forces in the determination of the leader's interpersonal style. There is nothing new about these feelings, for Thomas Jefferson knew of them in 1824. In a letter to Henry Lee, he wrote, "Men by their constitution are naturally divided into two parties: those who fear and distrust the people, and wish to draw all powers from them into the higher classes, and those who identify themselves with the people, have confidence in them, cherish and consider them as the most honest and safe, although not the most wise, depository of the public interest." Douglas McGregor's classic work on Theory X and Theory Y covered philosophical ground very similar to Jefferson's [13]. A leader who perceives subordinates to be untrustworthy, uncommitted, and unmotivated will seek to maintain close control and direction of the organization, to retain all the power and authority within the organization for himself, and to apply this power and authority unhesitatingly to accomplish goals and objectives.

The pattern of submissiveness that management-by-fear leaders demand may allow an organization to function, but it seems to be a dangerous characteristic in a health care institution where unstructured situations literally involving life and death arise everyday. Health care institutions need vigorous, flexible, self-starting staffs, not timid, rigid, tentative ones.

When a leader's life thrust has been to obtain a position of power and control, it is difficult to share decision making with subordinates and to encourage self-expression within the organization. These freedoms have a tendency to erode the leader's status and position, so some leaders cling to management-by-fear methods of control and motivation [14].

Coupled with fear of losing control is the fact that a disproportionate number of management-by-fear leaders are insensitive to people's feelings, again because of personal traits of the leader. Some people, for example, may pursue management careers to obtain power over others as a way of psychologically compensating for real or feared personal inadequacies, or as a reaction to an unconscious sense of helplessness. Their single-minded, perpetual pursuit of control blinds them to their own subtle feelings and those of others [15].

As a result of the complex interaction of all these factors, such leaders simply do not understand the power of people's feelings in the organizational environment. Nor do such leaders understand the powerful ways in which their oppressive leadership style alters the productivity of the people who work for them.

SUCCESSFUL LEADERSHIP

The key to successful leadership today is supportiveness. Leaders who can express respect for subordinates, show tolerance for honest mistakes made in the pursuit of organizational goals, and place trust and confidence in subordinates are practicing supportiveness. For many leaders this is a "natural" process and requires little effort on their part. Such leaders inherently believe that people are basically enthusiastic, like to work, are generally ambitious, are intelligent, and will accept responsibility for doing a job. (This is Douglas McGregor's Theory Y [16].)

The leader who exhibits a supportive leadership style can achieve a broad competence rather than restricted competence in his organization. This broader competence focuses on emphasizing individual growth, a willingness to execute assigned responsibility, experimentation that leads to progressive improvements, a striving toward autonomy, and conducting operations with as few predetermined rules and policies as rationality permits. This kind of organization leads to positive motivation over the long run, prepares subordinates for future roles of increased responsibility and authority, and is highly effective in obtaining short-run objectives [17]. A health care institution leader who is supportive produces a responsible, flexible staff that can function well under pressure. Modern health institutions can do with no less, and it is up to the leaders to make it happen.

A supportive leader understands and responds to the needs of subordinates. Health care personnel have the same basic needs as anyone else, and they bring their needs with them to the workplace. These needs, or motives, cause the people in the organization to engage in behavior to obtain satisfaction of these needs. Maslow categorized the needs that are common to all people as physiological, safety, social, self-esteem, and self-actualization needs [18]. Leaders who understand these needs can use the purposeful activity of their people to work toward organizational goals, obtaining in the proc-

ess satisfaction for both the needs of the people and the objectives of the organization. Management-by-fear leaders, since they do not understand these needs, often attempt to block the behavior of people that is directed toward need satisfaction in the organizational setting. When need-satisfying behavior is blocked, a process of frustration and alienation begins. If this process is not reversed, the effectiveness of the hospital is certain to be adversely affected.

Supportive leaders understand how human psychological needs impact day-to-day behavior of people in organizations. Devising control systems, writing policies and rules, developing organization structures, conducting interpersonal affairs, and a myriad of other elements of the administrator's job should be accomplished with these needs in mind. Through an understanding and appreciation of the behavioral impact of human needs, the motivations that are common to all people are channeled into patterns that are constructive for the organization. If the needs of people in the workplace are ignored or not understood, as happens in the management-by-fear style, then leadership of the organization will tend to frustrate satisfaction of needs, and people will channel their motive-satisfying behavior into patterns that are not constructive for the organization, especially in the long run.

HUMAN RELATIONS "LESSONS"

Supportive leaders practice constructive kinds of interpersonal relations. They have learned and internalized the results of countless thousands of bits of research and experimentation in human relations in organizations. This human relations experience and research has identified the kinds of leader behavior that are productive over the long run. Basically, analysis of human relations in organizations has shown that:

1. **Leaders must be sensitive to feelings of personal worth and human dignity in the subordinate.** Here is perhaps the underlying reason why the tongue-lashings of the management-by-fear leaders are so destructive: they are an affront to feelings of personal worth and human dignity.

2. **Leaders must take a personal interest in subordinates.** People need to be recognized, to be appreciated, to be understood. This requires an effort on the part of the hospital administrator, for he or she often has many subordinates, but it is a regarding endeavor. Sincerity is the key factor here. Insincere displays of personal interest retard rather than aid positive motivation. If an administrator cannot sincerely take a personal interest in other people, that administrator is miscast in a leadership role.

3. **Leaders must be open in communications with subordinates.** A leader must inform subordinates of those things about the organization—its objectives, policies, problems, prospects—which subordinates need to know to perform effectively within the organization. In the hospital setting, an open communication style becomes a particularly useful tool for coordinating the efforts of the diverse groups under the administrator's responsibility.

4. **Leaders must listen to their subordinates.** A leader must encourage open communications from subordinates. In this way the leader can build confidence, solve problems, and continually work on the building of a positive motivational environment. A two-way communications process is vital to hospital administrators, who encounter many situations in the trustee-administrator-physician organization structure where they are not in a position to utilize formal authority to achieve results, even if inclined to do so.

5. **Leaders must give subordinates an opportunity for participation in the organiza-** tion, through planning, directing, and controlling of their individual jobs. This is critical to building a commitment to organizational goals, which can seldom be accomplished by money alone. Money usually buys—induces—people to be members of an organization; it does not normally motivate them once a member. A sense of identity with the job does motivate people to give their best. If the job offers a chance for growth, recognition, achievement, promotion, and personal satisfaction, then the subordinate will seek self-control and self-responsibility. Overcontrol or overdirection is seldom beneficial in any organizational setting, but for the hospital administrator who is not sensitive to the needs of the nurse, technician, and paraprofessional groups, not to mention the physicians, to have a high degree of participation will encounter great difficulty.

Adopting these human relations "lessons" into their behavior pattern is not something management-by-fear leaders can do easily. They must be prepared to make significant changes in basic organization behavior. As William F. Whyte wrote, "The manager who hopes, by adding a technique or two to his repertoire, to introduce important changes in human relations, is only deluding himself. He won't fool others for very long" [19].

Our supervisor, after receiving the call from the family, might have positively supported the new head nurse by investigating the situation. She might have considered that the new head nurse was overwhelmed with learning to manage staff—or that a crisis had occurred to distract staff at the time of the patient's discharge—or that the family was anxious about taking the patient home. Open communication with the new head nurse might have revealed that person's needs for assistance in learning to handle events. The event, instead of producing anx-

iety, might have begun a helping, collaborative relationship to stimulate the head nurse's growth.

As the delivery of health care becomes more and more sophisticated, hospitals are employing more and more "knowledge workers." The tasks of these employees, in Peter Drucker's terminology, primarily involve implementation of knowledge through a physical act [20]. One finds a vast preponderance of knowledge workers in reviewing hospital occupational specialties. Drucker maintains that the knowledge worker will not produce if managed under Theory X assumptions about human nature. He says the knowledge worker has to be self-directed and wants to assume responsibility.

Fear is altogether incompatible with the production of knowledge work. While fear produces efforts, it also produces anxieties and will not produce results over the long run. In anything that has to do with knowledge, fear will produce only resistance [21].

In the constant quest for greater productivity, cost containment, and higher quality health care, the administrator should first look at the impact of his or her leadership style on the organization. A management-by-fear style, which either drives people away from the organization or reduces their effectiveness if they remain, has to be a serious impediment to organizational effectiveness. A supportive style of leadership can be an invaluable asset to organizational effectiveness.

FILLING IN THE MATRIX: THE LEADER

The parts of the model emphasized in the second unit are the leader, the workplace, and the health care industry. Direct your thoughts to your leadership role in your workplace as you consider the following focal points in this unit.

1. Leadership was considered in relation to situations, to leadership styles, and to goals to be achieved, in Unit 1. Now consider your interaction within the workplace and with those you lead.

a. Describe your workplace. Is the organization bureaucratic and traditional or is it characterized by being nontraditional and organic, with emphasis on behaviors?

b. Describe the level of professional competence of those you lead; are the majority professionals or is the mix characterized by few professionals and more subprofessionals?

c. Taking your responses from (a) and (b), consider how the characteristics of the workplace, the level of professional competence of those you lead, and your own concept of leadership contribute to the following in terms of situational favorableness or of achieving your work goals:

i. Your leader–follower relationships

ii. The degree of task structure in your department

iii. Your position power

(You may use the Ohio State studies and Fiedler's contingency theories as a base for your responses.)

2. Are you a manager, a leader, or both? To gain further insight into your behaviors, match the following behaviors to your leadership, using A (always), U (usually), S (sometimes), and N (never) to indicate which of the following are characteristic of your behavior:

_____ *Is willing to take risks*

_____ *Uses "direct" communication*

_____ *Uncovers new issues*

_____ *Has impersonal attitude toward goals*

_____ *Integrates self with work*

_____ *Professional-self is different from work-self*

_____ *Limits choices*

_____ *Is conservative*

_____ *Solves problems practically*

_____ *Is sensitive to others' feelings and thoughts*

_____ *Relates to others according to work roles*

_____ *Uses delaying tactics*

_____ *Feels separated from the environment*

_____ *Uses indirect communication*

_____ *Is in harmony with the environment*

_____ *Identifies with the organization*

_____ *Stresses self rather than organization*

How do your responses compare to the behaviors that Zaleznik associates with leaders, and with behaviors he associates with managers?

3. Do you think that managers and leaders are different types of persons? Do managers have traits different from those of leaders? Do you think that managers relate to employees differently than leaders?

    a. Compare managers and leaders according to their functions in the following categories:

       i. Concern for the dignity of others
      ii. Ability to socialize others into the field
    iii. Exercise of power and control over others
      iv. Ethical values
       v. Self-esteem

b. Leader—and manager—both function to accomplish work through others. Consider how you influence those you lead or manage.

i. Do you have frequent contact with those you lead?

ii. How do you use the organizational structure to keep informed of events taking place in your area of responsibility?

iii. Do your feelings or intuitions accurately reflect the reactions and responses of those you lead to your leadership? To the organization?

iv. How do you let those you lead know how you perceive their work?

v. How visible are you in the organization?

vi. Describe the three most influential persons employed in the department that you head. What are their roles? How do they influence others? What is their relationship to you? How are they recognized in the organization?

4. One of the functions of leaders is to develop others in the organization. Consider in light of the following mental exercises how persons become socialized in the department you lead.

a. Suppose that an individual who you think has leadership potential accepts a position in your department. Rate the following items from 1, as high, to 4, as low, as the method you would prefer to use to develop that person's leadership potential.

	1	2	3	4

i. Assign another or act as mentor yourself

ii. Assign a joint responsibility with a peer

iii. Appoint as your special assistant

iv. Assign to work with a group of health professionals from different disciplines

b. The position of your assistant is vacant and you have four choices of appointment sources. Rate the choices from 1, as high, to 4, as low, as the method you would select

	1	2	3	4

i. Appoint someone you trust who is currently employed in the department

ii. Appoint the applicant with the highest degree earned to fill the position

iii. Select the person most highly recommended to you by one or more trusted peers employed in other agencies

iv. Allow a committee of persons from the department to make the selection

5. How do you feel about yourself as an employee of the organization? Use the following questions to consider the points emphasized in this unit's content and to explore your feelings.

   a. Respond to the following items rating each as S if you feel strongly, M if your feelings are moderate, W if your feelings are weak, and 0 if you do not experience the feelings.

1. _____ I feel intimidated by those in authority over me.

2. _____ I feel that excessive control is exercised over my department.

3. _____ The organization's goals are different from my professional goals and I feel inhibited.

4. _____ My sense of organizational identity is high and I am proud to be employed by the organization.

5. _____ When persons in the department I lead disagree with me, I tend to feel frustrated.

6. _____ My leadership is of good quality and I feel good about myself in my position.

7. _____ I feel that others in the department do not have the same values that I hold about nursing.

8. _____ I feel that my position gives me an opportunity to be creative and to accomplish.

9. _____ I feel important to my organization and to the staff.

   b. How do you think that those you lead would respond to these same items? What feedback do you have that enables you to predict their responses?

REFERENCES AND NOTES

1. Maslow, A. **Eupsychian Management**. Homewood, Ill.: Irwin-Dorsey, 1965, p. 45.
2. Maslow, A., 1965, p. 44.
3. Maslow, A., 1965, p. 47.
4. Burns, J.M. **Leadership**. New York: Harper & Row, 1978, p. 78.
5. Maslow, A., 1965, p. 48.
6. Rockefeller, J.D., 3rd. **The Second American Revolution**. New York: Harper & Row, 1973, p. 72.
7. Levitt, T. Management and the post industrial society. **The Public Interest**, p. 73, Summer, 1976.
8. Hoffmann, S. and Hoffmann, I. The will for grandeur: de Gaulle as political artist. **Daedalus**, p. 849, Summer, 1968.
9. Zaleznik, A., Dalton, G.W., and Barnes, L.B. **Orientation and Conflict in Career**. Boston: Division of Research, Harvard Business School, 1970, p. 316.
10. Zaleznik, A., Dalton, G.W., and Barnes, L.B., 1970, p. 294.
11. James, W. **Varieties of Religious Experience**. New York: Mentor Books, 1958.
12. Jack Hanley got there by selling harder. **Fortune**, Nov., 1976.
13. McGregor, D., **The Human Side of Enterprise**. New York: McGraw-Hill, 1960.
14. Levinson, H. Asinine attitudes toward motivation. **Harvard Business Rev.**, p. 70, Jan.–Feb., 1973.
15. Levinson, H. 1973.
16. McGregor, D., 1960.
17. Morse, J.J., and Lorsch, J.W. Beyond Theory Y. **Harvard Business Rev.**, p. 61, May–June, 1970.
18. Maslow, A.H. **Motivation and Personality**, New York: Harper and Brothers, 1954, pp. 80–106.
19. Whyte, W.F. The Manipulation Problem. In Sayles, L.R. (Ed.) **Individualism and Big Business**. New York: McGraw-Hill, 1963.
20. Drucker, P.F. **Management: Tasks, Responsibilities, Practices**. New York: Harper & Row, 1974, p. 30.
21. Drucker, P.F., 1974, p. 241.

UNIT 3   LEADERSHIP
IN ORGANIZATIONS

In this Unit we will explore the interaction of the leader with the environmental components of our leadership model. We will focus on the environment of organizations and organizational behavior. The profession of nursing is concerned with providing a service that is in the public interest. The majority of nurses are employed by health care organizations or educational institutions that are subject to legislative action, external controls imposed on the health care industry, and community influences. Consequently there is considerable interaction among the workplace, the professional organization, and the individual's life about overlapping issues. The workplace defines and provides the service; the professional organization works to explicate a universal perception of the professional roles and the services; and each person is a consumer of the services. The issues of service overlap but are perceived from different viewpoints depending on the special interests of people in each component of the environment.

The workplace personnel are concerned with what is happening in the profession since professional activities deal with issues that can change or strengthen or threaten the provision of services that is the workplace's mission. Likewise, the profession is concerned with the functions and activities of people in the workplace because actual practice solidifies, weakens, defines, impedes, or stimulates professional practice. Finally, the nurse is a consumer of the services provided by the workplace and shares the public interest concerns for sanctioning the profession, for receiving the services the consumer as patient wants or desires, for ensuring continuity of services that are cost effective and practical. At the same time, the nurse draws monetary rewards necessary for goods and services that sustain life and that affect his or her quality of life in exchange for professional services rendered him or her as an employee in the workplace. Let us further explore the nature of the interaction of the leader by expanding some of these concepts.

*Large numbers of nurses in active practice are employees; few of the total number of practicing nurses are self-employed. What does it mean to be an employee? What is the value of employees to an organization? To explore these questions it is interesting to use age-old definitions of words to clarify current meanings. To **employ**, for example, is defined in Bailey's Universal Etymological English Dictionary (1801) as, "To set one at work; or about some business; to make use of." An organization employs nurses to set them at work; about the business of giving patient care, making use of the nurse's knowledge and skill.*

*Let us look at two more words from the same dictionary. The first, **organical** is defined (among naturalists) as "that part of a living creature or plant which is designed for the Performance of some particular Function or Action." An **organization** is defined as "The forming of organs, or instrumental parts." Nurses are among the professionals who are organical in an organization and nurses have a "particular Function or Action." In this respect we speak of the nurses' roles and functions. The instrumental parts of an organization are people, supplies, materials, machines, buildings, and equipment. The structure of the organization is the forming of organs. Each organizational structure places people in an orderly arrangement designed to facilitate their efficient functioning. How the organization is structured influences the relationships of people within that organization.*

Many health care agencies, particularly hospitals, are based on long-standing tradition. Many have long histories and are steeped in traditional bureaucratic organizational concepts and corresponding perceptions of the roles of personnel. Some health care agencies, such as health maintenance organizations (HMOs), are designed to revise the methods for delivery of health care. They are being formed to accommodate health care needs of the public that are not met by traditional hospital delivery systems. Some hospitals operate HMOs, indicating that traditional structures can change in response to newly defined needs thought to be in the public interest. Hospital organizations and HMOs are two examples of agencies in the health care industry. In comparing the two types of organizational structures, it is evident that the structure in which nurses, or any other professional group, function affects the action of the parts of the total organization. Similarly, the organizational structure affects how professionals function in these organizations.

There are many variations in organizations and their structures may be different according to the size and complexity of the organization, the relationships to the community, and the organization's purpose, goals, and values. Health care agencies are generally labor-intensive organizations, which means that people constitute the largest single resource used to produce services.

Health care agencies are also service-oriented organizations because their mission is to provide a public service that is sanctioned by societal mechanisms such as by charter, accreditation, consumer use, and community participation, to name a few [1–3]. While the organization is the forming of instrumental parts, the people employed by the organization select the music, tune the instruments, schedule the performances, and conduct the "integrated" playing of the instruments. All of these people have leaders who either emerge informally, or who are officially appointed by the organization.

Leadership then, is one aspect of organizational behavior. In service-oriented, labor-intensive organizations, leadership becomes a prominent concern. The organization is concerned with the leadership because leaders greatly influence how people are "set to work" or are "made use of." Employees are concerned with leadership for the same reasons. One difference is that the organization as an entity needs leadership to produce services while the individual needs leadership to ensure that his or her talents are made use of in appropriate ways that allow the person to go about his or her business effectively. When all of the people who are employed perceive that their business is congruent with the organization's expectations of their work, it can be surmised that both the individual and the organization are in harmony and are productive. Is this utopia? How does leadership function to achieve this type of congruence? Or can this congruence be achieved?

Lack of congruence between an employee's goals and the organization's goals can stem from many different sources. On one level, there can be differences in perceptions of goals that stem from the nature of manager-employee relationships. In one of the foregoing selections, for example, self-esteem was cited as critical for both leaders and those being led. The emphasis on one's own self-esteem and building self-esteem in others may seem idealistic to nurse-leaders who are in management positions. Those who are experiencing turmoil and conflict in their organizations and who are dealing with crisis intervention requiring expedient action may find it impossible to be sensitive to the feelings of employees. Such leaders are forced by circumstances to focus on accomplishing the activities demanded by the crisis situations. They are under duress to accomplish all the managerial work that seems necessary and simply may not have enough energy to deal with behaviors expected of leaders, the human development of employees, or even to listen to them well. As a result, employees may perceive a lack of congruence in their personal goals and those of the organization because their feelings are not heard or heeded sufficiently.

Another basic issue in leadership determining the congruence of an employee's goals with those of the organization centers on pro-

fessional autonomy. The degree of autonomy that nurses exercise in health care agencies varies. This variation in levels of autonomy can be traced to the diversity of types of administration in hospitals, to the attitudes of those in administrative roles in hospitals, to the scope of services provided by the hospitals, the size and complexity of the hospitals, and to the mix of personnel in the hospital, and to the nurses' perspective of their roles and functions [4–6]. In the present time, there is concern about threats to autonomy in the internal administration of services within hospitals [7–10]. Administrators, as professionals, are subject to external controls by state planning groups, federal intervention through grants and legislation, quality assurance programs, unions, and many other sources of external control. Nurses who are working in health care agencies are experiencing the effects of these increasing external controls. The question is: what happens to professional autonomy and to the services provided by care givers when external controls are increased?

Professional autonomy is an underlying theme of many changes in nursing education and nursing practice. It should be noted that professional autonomy does not just happen, but requires concerted effort by the professionals themselves. Because the majority of active nurses are employed by organizations, professional autonomy has to be nurtured within the context of institutional structures as well as within professional organizations and within the professionals themselves (11–13]. It becomes evident that nurse-leaders must balance the goals of achieving professional autonomy for nursing with the goals of the organizations that employ them and with their own perspective of their professional roles. The nurse-leader has the task of working with others in an organization in such a way that his or her professional goals contribute to the health and effectiveness of the organization as a whole. This task usually requires enlightenment of others in the organization about nursing's functions and their value to the organization.

As the educational level of nurses increases, the leader in nursing will relate to increasing numbers of nurses whose functions are dependent on sophisticated and autonomous application of knowledge. The leaders of these nurses will have to accommodate autonomy and independent decision making while developing networks of communication different from those of traditional organizational structures. This change contrasts vividly with the former emphasis on performance of task-oriented functions in nursing, which require a clear chain of command as determined by the traditional patterns of work assignment for nurses.

Nursing leaders in educational institutions have begun to deal with the impact of "knowledge workers" in the nursing field since they are dealing with an academically prepared group of people.

Leaders in nursing practice settings are just beginning to experience the impact of managing knowledge workers with advanced experience and academic preparation. Nursing leaders in the practice setting are being creative in increasingly actualizing the power of nursing knowledge in patient care by changing patterns of work assignment, changing job designs, changing the organizational structures, and thereby changing expectations of the nurse's function [14–15]. Concomitant with these changes is the trend to changing the mix of nursing personnel toward an increasingly professional staff.

While the nursing work force remains diverse in terms of educational preparation of its members, there is a definite, however gradual increase in the numbers of nurses with advanced education [16–18]. The advent of the doctor of nursing science degree and the increasing number of nurses with specialized education at the masters level is creating a need to change the perspectives of leadership as well as management in nursing. The leadership of the diversely prepared work force, in which there have been few "professionals" in the academic sense, is different from leadership that will be needed for a largely professional work force.

Nursing, in its struggle toward professional recognition, has generally supported increased education for nurses. Nonetheless, employment opportunities that realize the potential of these highly educated nurses are not always available. Nurse-leaders then have a two-fold problem. Not only must they work to change institutional perspectives of nursing roles and functions, but during the transition phase, when the lack of sufficient jobs to match their educational preparation causes nurses to accept employment in positions that do not fully tap their capabilities, the nurse-leaders must try to avert their employees' job dissatisfaction. The basic issue for leaders is how to promote job satisfaction for the knowledge worker within an organizational structure.

The leader may experience a conflict in loyalties—to the profession and to the workplace—when dealing with issues of professional autonomy. Some degree of congruence is important since nurses have a vested interest in all three components of the environment: the profession, their workplace, and the quality of their own lives. Nurses must be interested in the "welfare and quality of their workplace" for two very good reasons. One is that the quality of their employment depends on the stability of the workplace. The other reason is that nurses perform their functions and carry out their roles within organizations in such a way that their behaviors are an integrated part of the organizational behavior of the employing agency. The question is whether the organizational loyalties can be synonymous to the nurse's professional loyalties. In utopia they would be. In reality, these loyalties have the po-

tential for conflicting. Are you experiencing a conflict in loyalties? How do you support the development of the professional goals of nursing while supporting the organization in which you work?

Loyalties are charged with emotion and issues concerned with loyalties can easily become clouded by emotionality. Nursing is subject to many types of emotional conflict stemming from differences in opinion and theories among nurses, and between nurses and other persons or groups. The diversity in both nursing care delivery and in nursing education exemplifies emotion-laden policy issues. The diversity makes it difficult for nurses to portray the profession or to present the profession's values and attributes with clarity in the public domain. Confusion then results among consumers of nursing services, students who wish to enter nursing programs, employers of nurses, and legislators who are formulating public policy.

One way of reducing this confusion is to make nursing homogenous; this would require increasing homogeneity both in the delivery systems and in educational programs. Homogeneity in organizations within a broad system such as education or health care can lead to uniform management and decision-making systems. Nurses have not, however, demonstrated a willingness to become homogeneous in nursing practice or in education. Even though increasing uniformity in educational systems and in patterns of care administration can serve to reduce public confusion about nursing, there is a certain loss of freedom associated with loss of diversity. Some important questions to be considered in this regard include the following. Will the lessening of diversity in nursing educational programs improve the public understanding and consequently the public support of such programs? Is imagination impeded in a uniform system, or does imaginative and creative leadership require the nurturing of a diverse system? How are concepts of professional autonomy related to diversity?

Work-related pressures and the striving toward autonomy are two issues in nursing leadership in organizations. Both require that the leader step away from the milieu to reflect on values and goals, to determine his or her position in the organization, and to formulate strategies for future action. Developing a mental attitude and plan for future activities helps the leader deal more constructively with daily events as well as long-term activities. Because not every event can be planned, leaders must often deal with happenings that cannot be accurately forecasted. The future can, however, be shaped to a large degree by thoughtful and progressive planning. Good leaders are both present- and future-oriented, and have a sense of the meaning of the past. They must analyze the conflicts they are experiencing, use their opportunities, make decisions, recognize and use their power, and take action that resolves these conflicts constructively for the present and which shapes a desirable future.

The readings selected for this unit present a variety of viewpoints about leadership behaviors in organizations. Chester Barnard's chapter, "The Environment of Decision" is excerpted as the first selection. Barnard differentiates between personal and organizational decision making. The nurse-leader who has accepted a management position in an organization also accepts the responsibility for participating in organizational decision making. The nurse-manager represents one part of the organization; the part concerned with nursing is a significant portion of a health care agency. The aggregate contribution to organizational decision making is more effective if persons representing each part of the organization participate strongly, offering opinions and advice that represent the sound professional practice in their area of work and expertise. If everyone participates, organizational decisions can better support both the organization's welfare and the professional practice of member groups such as nurses.

Using the distinction made earlier between management and leadership, one can analyze the occasions for decision cited by Barnard. Those originating from authoritative communication from superiors and those referred by subordinates belong in the realm of management. Those originating in the initiative of the executive belong in the realm of leadership. The nurse-leader who is a manager, however, interprets and defines the means–ends decisions from the perspective of nursing for decisions arising from "all occasions" and thus can promote professional autonomy in management in all decision making. In those decisions initiated by the nurse-leader, the professional autonomy is exercised with far greater visibility. Because the services provided by health care agencies are patient-care services, nursing can and should initiate decisions within an organization. The "specialty" of nursing is the focus of the organization's service, patient care.

Barnard speaks of making decisions as planning; he refers to the need to make sense of a complex environment. The latter point may remind you of a point I made in the introduction, that the leader can select the terrain over which he or she will pass—in fact the leader-manager often charts out the terrain, thus providing direction for others. In so doing, nurse-leaders realize the need for competence in making decisions. When working with specialized knowledge workers such as professional nurses, the leader may find that his or her own competence is insufficient (a decision-making factor cited by Barnard). This is a dilemma of managers of knowledge workers that must be accepted and resolved. Collaboration and consultation with the specialized knowledge workers is necessary to produce effective decisions. Another aspect of deci-

sion making pertinent for nurse-leaders that Barnard cites is that certain decision-making capabilities of subordinates can be taken for granted. In nursing, if nurses are professionals and autonomous, the leader or manager can realistically expect that they not only are capable of making decisions but also need to be given the prerogatives of professional decison making.

Making decisions is one way of using power. The next selection, another portion of the chapter by Fred Luthans that was excerpted in Unit 1, is an exploration of the meaning of dynamics of power. Nurse-leaders function within organizations from a power base of both personal and organizational power. This power, like leadership, to which it is closely related, is difficult to explain. Luthans, however, writes about the relation between power and leadership with clarity and from a broad perspective that includes consideration of groups, conflict, and motivation.

Of particular interest to nurses seeking professional autonomy is "expert power." Leaders of nurses who recognize the correlation of expert power with satisfaction and performance can adapt their leadership behaviors accordingly. Are you secure enough in your personal life, in your profession, and in your workplace to let others exercise their "expert power?" It can be considered that "security" of individuals in this regard is a necessary basis for the aggressive interchange required within nursing to resolve conflicts and to shape the future.

Another dimension of making decisions relates to the environment in our model. Nurses, like other professionals, continually negotiate the terms of their practice with the profession, the workplace, and their personal lives. Leaders negotiate the boundaries of their roles and also negotiate change. Negotiation involves decision making. In fact, how one makes decisions is part of broader interaction processes that take place both within and outside of organizations.

A clever introduction to negotiation appears in a book about the topic written by Anselm Strauss. To quote:

Negotiate — bargain, contract, arrange

Bargain — negotiate, contract

Contract — agreement, bargain, arrangement

Agreement — accord, reconcilement, understanding, contract, compact

Compact — contract, settlement, bargain, negotiation, arrangement, understanding

Understanding — compact, agreement, adjustment

Adjustment — reconcile, settle, arrange

Reconcile — adjust, settle

Settle — reconcile, fix, stabilize (see arrangement)

Arrangement — settle, organize, coordinate, orderliness

Coordinate — adjust, organize

Organize — arrange, coordinate, systematize

Systematize — arrange, organize, coordinate

Order — arrangement, systematization [19]

From the Introduction, *Negotiations: Varieties, Contexts, Processes, and Social Order* **by Anselm Strauss. Published by Jossey Bass, 1978. Reprinted with permission.**

One of the functions of a negotiator is to bring others to a certain perspective or point of view through interaction. Leaders in organizations have, as one of their functions, to negotiate in order to "enlighten" the people who work in the organization about changing nursing practice. Being concerned for the future and paving the way for change is an attribute of a leader, as well as of an organization.

The next selection in this unit was written by June Werner, who expresses the view that decision making, power, and leadership are related to enlightenment of others in an organization. She presents a model of how nurse-leaders can initiate decisions at all levels of an organization to make not only nursing but the organization more effective. One may ask how nursing leaders are to accomplish this enlightenment. Does the leader's commitment to initiating and developing changes in institutional perspectives require charisma? Does it depend on expert negotiation skills? Is it a function of excellent decision making? Or is it the product of competence in the nursing staff? Whichever the answer, we might agree that it is a function of leadership, and that the leader not only is motivated to succeed personally but also is motivated to make the workplace succeed. Maslow writes:

The managers of any enterprise want it to continue and they don't mean for two or three years, they mean for fifty years or a hundred years. And not only do they want it to continue for a hundred years (which makes necessary, then, the profoundest discussion of human motives and human far goals), but they would also like their organism, the group or the enterprise, or the organization to grow in a healthy way. [20]

Nurse-leaders work with groups of other nurses and different professionals to maintain the growth of organizations. One important function of leaders in this capacity is the organizational use of power and decision making to formulate policy. J. M. Burns writes about decisions made by leaders in formulating policy:

Typically leaders as policy makers operate in relatively settled and even structured political situations, within broadly agreed on boundaries and constraints, governed by established and legitimating traditions, precedents, and pronouncements. Party leaders act within the mythology of popular heroes and symbols, party platforms and procedures, external competition and internal pressure. Legislative leaders respond to constitutional and political restraints and opportunities. Judicial policy makers take account of statutes and precedents that, even in their ambiguous and contradictory legitimations, establish directions and guidelines. In a relatively stable political system leaders will also be bound by their own previous commitments. [21]

Earlier in this anthology it was stated that nursing needs leaders to shape the future. Consider the decisions you make that become policy. Do you maintain the status quo? Or do you initiate change through policy formulation rather than follow precedent? What commitments do you have? Are you bound by restraints? Are these restraints perceived or real? What statutes or traditions do you invoke? What are your conflicts? Do they stem from the intersection of internal and external pressures? What events in your organization stimulate your decisions? What guidelines and information govern your decisions?

Leaders need more information to make decisions and those who are managers in organizations obtain much of their information about operations from the persons they lead or manage. "Leadership, Learning, and Changing the Status Quo," written by Chris Argyris, is included here to explicate how the person in charge can find out the "truth" about operations in the nursing organization and, in the process, facilitate both self-growth and development of employees. Implicit in this growth is developing the autonomy of individuals—an issue predominant in nursing. Emphasis on professional autonomy may remain verbiage in nursing literature unless the leaders and managers construct systems and patterns of care delivery in which nurses are not only responsible—a value long held by the profession—but also autonomous in making decisions in their realm of practice. Argyris' theme of learning in organizations supports use of participative leadership styles described in Unit 1.

Even effective leaders experience conflict and ambivalence in their leadership roles. Despite high self-esteem and belief in the future, periods of self-questioning are inevitable. Merton's essay is included to illustrate that these feelings are normal for leaders. "The Ambivalence of Organizational Leaders: An Interpretative Essay," realistically describes some of the conflicts of leaders. Merton supports the hypotheses that leadership is concerned with social interaction, that leadership styles vary, and that leaders in organizations are concerned with the welfare of the total organiza-

tion. His ending sentence should be read before beginning study of the essay: *"And still the question remains, How shall leaders of organizations steer their course through the ambivalences and contradictions of leadership? What concepts shall they use as their guide?"*

The final article in this unit deals with leadership development in organizations. The current status of health care organizations represents a point in the evolution of management and the health care organization; one can find certain theories in this historical development that have taken hold and have continued to be predominant in organizational practices in certain settings. Nurses in leadership roles in organizations have the power to determine whether these historical practices should be perpetuated or changed.

Some critical issues for nurse-leaders in organizations are dealt with. What is the relation between morale and productivity? Is a human relations management model less rational than a bureaucratic management model? How does a leader integrate professional and organizational goals? What types of work values are inculcated in nursing students during their nursing education? Are these values in conflict with those of the workplace? Bennis writes that core organizational problems and tasks are integration, social influence, collaboration, adaptation, and revitalization [22]. How can nurses be socialized so that they will make a commitment to dealing with the core organizational problems and tasks? Finally, how can nurses learn the fine art of negotiation? Exercising leadership to resolve some of these issues is challenging.

Resolution of these issues and integration of professional and organizational goals depends on several activities. First, nurses must demonstrate through their day-by-day practice how their functions contribute to and develop organizational goals. Second, together all nurses in society must formulate realistic goals for their profession in terms of standards of care, educational preparation for given areas of practice, and role interpretations that support changing and evolving nursing practice. Third, nurses must continually negotiate with other health professionals and legislators to determine how the role of the nurse should evolve. Fourth, nurses must make a commitment to the nurses' roles and functions and must maintain control over all aspects of these functions. Finally, nurses must learn to communicate constructively with others to interpret the profession to the public.

There are many nurses who devote much time and energy to accomplishing these several activities. The long-term future of nursing as a profession, however, depends on socialization of every nurse in a "professional perspective." The practicing nurse contributes the most significant impetus toward the development of the profession by acting like a professional in everyday practice. Nurse-leaders who emerge from groups of nurses in active practice help to support this professional function by interpreting nursing in planning-groups, in the development of ways and means to facilitate professional practice, and in communicating professional responses and needs to society. The actions of these leaders lose credibility in society, however, when they are different from the actual practice of nursing or when the perspectives of the leaders are different from the perspectives of those who are in active practice. All nurses employed by health care organizations must have a part in the processes of developing and interpreting their profession both in the organization and in the public.

To conclude this anthology, consider the many important issues in nursing and some ways we can shape the future of our profession. Can nursing tolerate ambiguity? How should nurses collaborate to solve their problems of a professional nature? How can nursing be better integrated into health care organizations from both management and leadership perspectives? Finally, how can nurses best participate in the profession's social evolution? Who will our leaders be and where will they take us? What quality of life can we nurses expect in our future?

THE ENVIRONMENT OF DECISION

By Chester I. Barnard

The acts of individuals may be distinguished in principle as those which are the result of deliberation, calculation, thought, and those which are unconscious, automatic, responsive, the results of internal or external conditions present or past. In general, whatever processes precede the first class of acts culminate in what may be termed "decision." Involved in acts which are ascribed to decision are many subsidiary acts which are themselves automatic, the processes of which are usually unknown to the actor.

When decision is involved there are consciously present two terms—the end to be accomplished and the means to be used. The end itself may be the result of logical processes in which the immediate end is in turn a means to some broader or more remote end. The ultimate end may not be a result of logical processes, but "given"—that is, unconsciously impressed—by conditions, including social conditions past or present, including orders of organizations. But whenever the end has been determined, by whatever process, the decision as to means is itself a logical process of discrimination, analysis, choice—however defective either the factual basis for choice or the reasoning related to these facts.

The acts of organizations are those of persons dominated by organizational, not personal, ends. These ends, especially the most general or remote, represent a consensus of opinion and may be arrived at by nonlogical processes; but since they must usually be formulated (whereas individual ends more rarely need to be formulated) the ends of organizations involve logical processes, not as rationalizations after decision but as processes of decision. Moreover, when ends have been adopted, the coordination of acts as means to these ends is itself an essentially logical process. The discrimination of facts and the allocation of acts by specialization which coordination implies may quite appropriately be regarded as logical or deliberate thinking processes of organization, though not necessarily logical processes of thought of the individual participants. The more important **organization** acts of individuals are likely to be logical—in that they require deliberate choice of means to accomplish ends which are not personal, and therefore cannot be directly automatic or responsive reactions.

It is the deliberate adoption of means to ends which is the essence of formal organization. This is not only required in order to make cooperation superior to the biological powers and senses of individuals, but it is possibly the chief superiority of cooperative compared to individual action in organizations.

From this analysis it follows that acts of decision are characteristic of organizational behavior as contrasted with individual behavior.

The formulation of organizations' purposes or objectives and the more general decisions involved in this process and in those of action to carry them into effect are distributed in organizations, and are not, nor can they be, concentrated or specialized to individuals except in minor degree.

Every effort that is a constituent of organization, that is, every coordinated cooperative effort, may involve two acts of decision. The first is the decision of the person affected as to whether or not he will contribute this effort as a matter of personal choice. It is a detail of the process of repeated personal decisions that determine whether or not the individual will be or will continue to be a contributor to the organization.

The second type of decision views the effort concerning which decision is to be made nonpersonally, from the viewpoint of its effect on the organization and of its relation to the organization's purpose. This second act of decision is often made in a direct sense by individuals, but it is impersonal and organizational in its intent and effect. Very often it is also organizational in its process, as, for example, in legislatures, or when boards or committees determine action. The act of decision is a part of the organization itself.

These two kinds of decision—organizational decisions and personal decisions—are chiefly to be distinguished as to process by this fact: that personal decisions cannot ordinarily be delegated to others, whereas organizational decisions can often if not always be delegated. For example, what may

be called a major decision by an individual may require numerous subsidiary decisions (or judgments) which he also must make. A similar important decision by an organization may in its final form be enunciated by one person and the corresponding subsidiary decisions by several different persons, all acting organizationally, not personally. Similarly, the execution of a decision by one person may require subsequent detailed decision by him as to various steps, whereas the execution of a similar decision in an organization almost always requires subsequent detailed decision by several different persons. Indeed, it may be said that often the responsibility for an organizational decision is not a personal responsibility until assigned. Responsibility for organizational decision must be assigned positively and definitely in many cases because the aptness of a decision depends upon knowledge of facts and of the organization's purpose, and is therefore bound up with organizational communication.

An organization imposes the assignment of responsibility for some kinds of organizational decision to executives. A characteristic of the services of executives is that they represent a specialization of the process of making organizational decisions—and this is the essence of their functions.

The executive must distinguish between the occasions for decision in order to avoid the acceptance of more than he can undertake without neglecting the fields to which his position relates. For the natural reluctance of other men to decide, their persistent disposition to avoid responsibility, and their fear of criticism will lead them to overwhelm the executive who does not protect himself from excessive burdens of decision if he is not already protected by a well-regulated and habitual distribution of responsibilities.

It is necessary in the making of decisions to maintain a balance between the fields from which the occasions of them arise. The occasions for decision originate in three distinct fields: 1) from authoritative communications from superiors; 2) from cases referred for decision by subordinates; 3) from cases originating in the initiative of the executive concerned.

1. Occasions for decision are frequently furnished by instructions or by general requirements of superior authority. Such decisions relate to the interpretation, application, and distribution of instructions. These occasions cannot be avoided, though the burden may be reduced by delegation of responsibility to subordinates. They involve serious decisions when the instructions seem morally wrong, harmful to the organization, or impossible of execution.

The nurse-manager is faced with this type of decision when interpreting or applying rules and regulations for federal grant participation, when determining the mix of nursing staff according to an allotted budget, or when supporting a staff nurse who questions a physician's order for a medication.

2. The cases referred for decision may be called appellate cases. They arise from incapacity of subordinates, uncertainty of instructions, novelty of conditions, conflict of jurisdiction or conflicts of orders, or failure of subjective authority. The control of the number of appellate cases lies in adequacy of executive organization, of personnel, of previous decision; and the development of the processes of informal organization. The test of executive action is to make these decisions when they are important, or when they cannot be delegated reasonably, and to decline the others.

Nurse-managers face this type of decision when negotiating to close beds when there is inadequate nursing staff, refusing to open a new special-care unit when nurses are not yet prepared to function in that specialty, when hearing personnel conflicts or solving problems of the relationship of nursing to supporting service departments.

3. The occasions for decision that arise on the initiative of the executive are the most important test of his capacity. Out of his understanding of the situation, which depends upon his ability and initiative, and on the character of the communication system of his organization, it is to be determined whether something needs to be done or corrected. To decide that question involves not merely the ordinary elements but the executive's specific justification for deciding. For when the occasions for decision arise from above or below the position of the executive, others have in advance granted him authority; but when made on his own initiative, this always may be (and generally is) questioned, at least tacitly (in the form whether decision was necessary, or related to scope of obligations, etc.). Moreover, failure to decide is usually not specifically subject to attack, except under extreme conditions. Hence there is much incentive to avoid decision. Pressure of other work is the usual self-justification. Yet it is clear that the most important obligation is to raise and decide those issues which no one else is in a position to raise effectively.

Nurse-managers face these decisions when determining the quality and essence of nursing care in an institution. Should there be an all RN staff, should nurses write nursing orders, should team-nursing patterns be changed to primary-nursing patterns—these are a few of the decisions that can be brought from the staff nurses or from the board.

From the point of view of the **relative** importance of specific decisions, those of executives properly call for first attention. From the point of view of **aggregate** importance, it is not decisions of executives but of nonex-

ecutive participants in organization which
should enlist major interest. Indeed it is
precisely for this reason that many executive
decisions are necessary—they relate to the
facilitation of correct action involving appropriate decision among others. In large
measure this is a process of providing for the
clear presentment of the issues or choices.
Coordination of action of the nonexecutive
participants in organization requires
repeated organizational decisions "on the
spot" where the effective action of organization takes place. It is here that the final and
most concrete objectives of purposes are
found, with the maximum of definiteness.
There is no further stage of organizational
action.

*Nurse-managers initiate many "auto-
matic" decisions among staff members when
making decisions about protocols or rules,
or acceptable practices. The nurse who
knows that the nurse-manager will support a
decision to obtain food for a hungry patient
at midnight will not stop to consider choices,
but will order the food. The action is accomplished.*

The types of decision as well as the conditions change in character as we descend from
the major executive to the nonexecutive positions in organization. At the upper limit
decisions relating to ends to be pursued
generally require the major attention, those
relating to means being secondary, rather
general, and especially concerned with personnel, that is, the development and protection of organization itself. At intermediate
levels the breaking of broad purposes into
more specific ends and the technical and
technological problems, including economic
problems, of action become prominent. At
the low levels decisions characteristically
relate to technologically correct conduct, so
far as the action is organization action. But
it is at these low levels, where ultimate

authority resides, that the **personal** decisions
determining willingness to contribute
become of relatively greatest aggregate importance.

*The director or leader determines the
organizational structure, the midlevel
managers implement the structure, and the
staff nurses give patient care within the
structure, choosing to support or not support the overall goals.*

THE EVIDENCES OF DECISION

Not the least of the difficulties of appraising
the executive functions or the relative merits
of executives lies in the fact that there is little
direct opportunity to observe the essential
operations of decision.

Those decisions which are most directly
known result in the authoritative communications, that is, orders. Something is or
is not to be done. Even in such cases the
basic decision may not be evident; for the
decision to attempt to achieve a certain result
or condition may require several communications to different persons which appear to be complete in themselves but in
which the controlling general decision may
not be disclosed.

Again, a firm decision may be taken that
does not result in any communication
whatever for the time being. A decision
properly timed must be made in advance of
communicating it, either because the action
involved must await anticipated developments or because it cannot be authoritative
without educational or persuasive preparation.

Finally, the decision may be not to decide.
This is a most frequent decision, and from
some points of view probably the most important. For every alert executive continually raises in his own mind questions for determination. As a result of his consideration he

may determine that the question is not pertinent. He may determine that it is not now pertinent. He may determine that it is pertinent now, but that there are lacking adequate data upon which to base a final decision. He may determine that it is pertinent for decision now, but that it should or must be decided by someone else on the latter's initiative. He may determine that the question is pertinent, can be decided, will not be decided except by himself, and yet it would be better that it be not decided because his competence is insufficient.

The fine art of executive decision consists in not deciding questions that are not now pertinent, in not deciding prematurely, in not making decisions that cannot be made effective, and in not making decisions that others should make. Not to decide questions that are not pertinent at the time is uncommon good sense, though to raise them may be uncommon perspicacity. Not to decide questions prematurely is to refuse commitment of attitude or the development of prejudice. Not to make decisions that cannot be made effective is to refrain from destroying authority. Not to make decisions that others should make is to preserve morale, to develop competence, to fix responsibility, and to preserve authority.

From this it may be seen that decisions fall into two major classes, positive decisions—to do something, to direct action, to cease action, to prevent action; and negative decisions, which are decisions not to decide. Both are inescapable; but the negative decisions are often largely unconscious, relatively nonlogical, "instinctive," "good sense." It is because of the rejections that the selection is good.

THE NATURE OF THE ENVIRONMENT

Whatever the occasions or the evidences of decision, it is clear that decisions are constantly being made. What is the nature of the environment of decisions, the materials with which they deal, the field to which they relate? It consists of two parts: 1) purpose; and 2) the physical world, the social world, the external things and forces and circumstances of the moment. All of these, including purpose, constitute the objective field of decision; but the two parts are of different nature and origin. The function of decision is to regulate the relations between these two parts. This regulation is accomplished either by changing the purpose or by changing the remainder of the environment.

1. We may consider purpose first. It may seem strange perhaps that purpose should be included in the objective environment, since purpose of all things seems personal, subjective, internal, the expression of desire. This is true; but **at the moment of a new decision,** an existing purpose, the result of a previous decision under previous conditions, is an objective fact, and it is so treated at that moment insofar as it is a factor in new decision.

This is especially true because organizational decisions do not relate to personal purposes, but to organizational purposes. The purpose which concerns an organizational decision may have been given as a fact to and accepted as such by the person who is responsible for making a new decision. But no matter how arrived at, when decision is in point, the purpose is fact already determined; its making is a matter of history; it may be as objective as another man's emotions may be to an observer.

In nursing leadership we must take care to prevent history from making current decisions. What is fixed might need to be changed. Decisions made in past environments may not be appropriate for present and future environments. The purposes

*of present decisions may be the same as for
past decisions but the new environment
places different interpretations on purpose.
What was good-quality patient care in 1902
is different from good-quality patient care in
1980 or 2000.*

Purpose itself has no meaning except in an
environment. It can only be defined in terms
of an environment. (Care should be taken to
keep in mind that environment throughout
does not mean merely physical aspects of the
environment, but explicitly includes social
aspects, although physical rather than other
aspects are used for illustration.) Even to
want to go somewhere, anywhere, supposes
some kind of environment. A very general
purpose supposes a very general undifferen-
tiated environment; and if the purpose is
stated or thought of it must be in terms of
that general environment. But when formed,
it immediately (if it is not in suspense or dor-
mant, so to speak) serves for reducing that
environment to more definite features; and
the immediate result is to change purpose into a more specific purpose. Thus when I
decide I want to go from A to B, my idea of
terrain is vague. But as soon as I have decided, the terrain becomes less vague; I immediately see paths, rocks, obstacles that are
significant; and this finer discrimination
results in detailed and smaller purposes. I
not only want to go from A to B, but I want
to go this way, that way, etc. This constant
refinement of purpose is the effect of
repeated decisions, in finer and finer detail,
until eventually detailed purpose is contem-
poraneous accomplishment. But similarly
with each new edition of purpose, a new
discrimination of the environment is involved, until finally the last obstacle of
progressive action represents a breaking up
of a general purpose into many concrete
purposes, each made almost simultaneously
with the action. The thing is done as soon as

decided; it becomes a matter of history; it
constitutes a single step in the process of
experience.

Thus back and forth purpose and environment react in successive steps through successive decisions in greater and greater
detail. A series of final decisions, each apparently trivial, is largely accomplished unconsciously and sums up into an effected
general purpose and a route of experience.

2. We may now consider the environment
of decision exclusive of purpose. It consists
of atoms and molecules, agglomerations of
things in motion, alive; of men and emotions; of physical laws and social laws; social
ideas, norms of action, of forces and
resistances. Their number is infinite and they
are all always present. They are also always
changing. They are meaningless in their
variety and changes except as discriminated
in the light of purpose. They are viewed as
static facts, if the change is not significant
from the viewpoint of the purpose, or as
both static and dynamic facts.

This discrimination divides the world into
two parts; the facts that are immaterial, irrelevant, mere background; and the part that
contains the facts that apparently aid or prevent the accomplishment of purpose. As
soon as that discrimination takes place, decision is in bud. It is in the state of selecting
among alternatives. These alternatives are
either to utilize favorable factors, to
eliminate or circumvent unfavorable ones,
or to change the purpose. Note that if the
decision is to deal with the environment, this
automatically introduces new but more
detailed purposes, the progeny, as it were, of
the parent purpose; but if the decision is to
change the purpose rather than deal with the
environment, the parent is sterile. It is abandoned, and a new purpose is selected,
thereby creating a **new** environment in the
light of **that** purpose.

The profession of nursing is undergoing many changes involving decisions of both purpose and environment. In nursing education efforts are being made to change the environment in which the education takes place. Likewise, efforts are being made to change the environment in which health care consumers receive care. The general purposes may remain stable—that is, education or patient care—but the new environmental variables have the effect of changing the specific purposes.

LEADERSHIP AND POWER
(an excerpt)

By Fred Luthans

THE MEANING AND DYNAMICS OF POWER

As indicated in the introductory comments of this chapter (see Unit 1), there is a close relation between leadership and power. Especially when leadership is defined as influencing others, much can be learned about leadership by understanding power, and vice versa. In the following paragraphs the meaning of power is examined, the sources and types of power are identified, and the use of power in organizations is analyzed.

The Meaning of Power

The power motive is defined as the need to manipulate others and have superiority over them. Given this definition of the need for power, power itself can be defined as an ability to get an individual or group to do something—to get the person or group to change in some way. The person who possesses power has the ability to manipulate or change others. Such a definition of power distinguishes it from authority and influence.

Authority legitimates power. Authority is the **right** to manipulate or change others. Power need not be legitimate. Influence is usually conceived as being narrower than power. It involves the ability on the part of a person to alter another person or group in specific ways, such as in their satisfaction and performance. Influence is more closely associated with leadership than is power, but both obviously are involved in the leadership process. Therefore, authority is different from power because of its legitimacy, and influence is narrower than power but is so conceptually close that the two terms can be used interchangeably.

The foregoing points out that an operational definition for power is lacking and, because of its vagueness, the concept of power has been largely ignored in the study of organizational behavior. Hicks and Gullett point out the problems with the study of power when they say, "Because power is not well understood, is often extremely subtle or obscure, springs from multiple sources, is highly dynamic, has multiple causes and effects, is multidimensional, and is particularly difficult—if not impossible—to quantify, positivists have tended to ignore it" [23]. Yet, by looking at the sources and types of power and the organizational use of it, much can be learned about leadership in particular and organizational behavior in general.

123

Sources and Types of Power

The most widely recognized categories of the sources of power come from French and Raven [24]. They identify the following bases of power:

1. **Reward power.** The person having this power has the ability to reward. Managers frequently have reward power in that they can give merit increases or incentive pay and promotions to their subordinates. In operant terms this means the person has the power to administer positive reinforcers. In expectancy terms this means that the person has the power to provide positive valences and the other person perceives this ability.

2. **Coercive power.** The person having this power has the ability to threaten and/or punish. Managers frequently have coercive power in that they can fire or demote subordinates or dock their pay. They can also directly or indirectly threaten an employee that these punishing consequences will occur. In operant terms this means the person has the power to administer punishment or to negatively reinforce (terminate punishing consequences, which is a form of negative control). In expectancy terms this means that power comes from the expectation on the part of the other persons that they will be punished if they will not conform to the powerful person's desires.

3. **Legitimate power.** This power stems from the internalized values of the other persons which give the legitimate right to the person to influence them. This, of course, could be labeled authority rather than power. The other persons have the obligation to accept this power. Such legitimate power can come from cultural values, acceptance of the social structure, or the designation of a legitimizing agent. Managers generally have legitimate power because employees believe in private property law and in the hierarchy where higher positions have been designated to have power over lower positions.

4. **Referent power.** This type of power comes from the feeling or desire on the part of the other persons to identify with the person wielding power. The other persons want to identify with the powerful person regardless of the outcomes. A manager who desires to have referent power must be attractive to subordinates so that they want to identify with the manager regardless of whether the manager gives rewards or punishment.

5. **Expert power.** Managers have expert power to the extent that the other employees attribute knowledge and expertise to them. The experts are seen to have knowledge or ability only in well-defined areas. In an organization engineers may have expert power in their area of specialization but not outside of it. For example, the engineers are granted power on production problems but not on personnel problems. The same holds true for other staff experts such as accountants and computer technologists.

French and Raven recognize that there may be other sources of power, but these are the major ones. They also point out that the five sources are interrelated (e.g., the use of coercive power by managers may reduce their referent power) and the same person may use different types of power under different circumstances and at different times.

Research on Power

There has been some research devoted to the French and Raven categories of power. Schopler reviewed several studies that directly tested the bases of power and found that coercive power induces greater resistance than reward power; users of reward power are liked better than those depending on coercive power; conformity to coercive power increases with the strength of the potential punishment; as the legitimacy of a punishing act increases, the conformity increases; and expertness on one task increases the ability to exert influence on a second task [25]. Schopler does point out that the interdependence of the bases of power may contaminate the findings.

Of more direct relevance to organizational behavior are the studies that have related the bases of a manager's power or control to satisfaction and performance. On the basis of five organizational studies (branch office, college, insurance agency, production work units, and utility company work group) the following conclusions were drawn on each of the French and Raven bases of power [26].

1. **Expert power** was most strongly and consistently correlated with satisfaction and performance.

2. **Legitimate power** along with expert power was rated as the most important basis of complying with a supervisor's wishes but was an inconsistent factor in organizational effectiveness.

3. **Referent power** was given intermediate importance as a reason for complying and in most cases was positively correlated with organizational effectiveness.

4. **Reward power** was also given intermediate importance for complying but had inconsistent correlations with performance.

5. **Coercive power** was by far the least prominent reason for complying and was actually negatively related to organizational effectiveness.

The conclusion from research so far is that **the nonformal bases of power (expert and referent)** impact most favorably on organizational effectiveness. However, such a conclusion should be interpreted with caution because, like the Likert studies, the studies on power are almost all based on questionnaire responses and may reflect the cultural values of the respondents instead of the actual uses of power in an organization.

The Use of Power in an Organization

The French and Raven bases of power point out that some types of power may have a positive impact on organizational effectiveness and others may not. In general, the research on power follows the findings in leadership styles reported earlier in the chapter. The important implication is that leadership and power approaches and uses can be good or bad for the organization.

In society as a whole, "power" generally has a negative connotation. The commonly used term **power hungry** reflects this negative feeling about power.

McClelland feels that negative use of power is associated with personal power. He feels that it is primitive and has negative consequences.

The contrasting other face of power is social power. It is characterized by a "concern for group goals, for finding those goals that will move men, for helping the group to formulate them, for taking some initiative in providing members of the group with the means of achieving such goals, and for giving group members the feeling of strength and competence they need to work hard for such goals" [27]. This social power points out that the leader is often in a precarious position, walking the fine line between exhibiting personal dominance and the more socializing use of power.

Power is inevitable in organizations. One of Adolf Berle's several "laws" of power is that power invariably fills any vacuum in human organization [28]. How power is used and what type of power is used will vitally affect organizational goals. In French and Raven's terms, the use of expert and referent power in organizations may be more effective than traditionally used legitimate and coercive power. In McClelland's terms, social power may be of greater value to the organization than is traditionally used personal power. Research gives some indication that such conclusions are valid. But once again, the use of the various types of power depends on the situation. Contingency models of power are needed. A challenge for the future will be to better understand power and how it is contingently related to varying situations.

WHAT IS NEEDED IN LEADERSHIP FOR NURSING ADMINISTRATION

By June Werner

Reprinted with permission from *Nursing Administration Quarterly*, Fall 1976. Published by Aspen Systems Corporation, Germantown, Maryland.

Who determines what constitutes success in nursing leadership? One of the problems is that many people in several disciplines make that very important decision. Each discipline is distinct, having separate and often dichotomous criteria for success in nursing leadership.

The successful leader in nursing must have skills which relate to all facets of administration. This includes development of a staff which will provide quality nursing care for patients and their families, planning and control of the personnel and fiscal aspects of the department, and the maintenance of effective relationships with the administrative staff and 20 to 30 other departments in the hospital.

We make the assumption that we function in the institution or agency in which we are employed as if it were an individual entity; that we are circumscribed by institutional values and standards and a singular set of rules, policies and just one value system. Leadership in nursing must accept the reality that though we may work for an institution or agency with one name, it is ultimately a conglomerate of separate cultures, each with its own values and standards.

If we were to examine just a few of the many separate cultures within a hospital we might look at the board of directors, the administrative staff, the physician group, the support departments, and the department of nursing, and possibly others. Four significant aspects of each of these five cultures are standards by which they can be measured: 1) those things they consider most important, 2) those things they fear, 3) their preconceived notions, and 4) their expectations of the nurse administrator. These are illustrated in Exhibit 3-1.

If the standards of these groups are as different as seen in the exhibit, we are obviously dealing with distinct cultures. What implications does this multifaceted cultural nature of a hospital have for a nursing administrator? First, she must interact effectively with each group (and with each significant individual within each group). Second, the nurse-administrator must present herself to each of these groups as an authentic, confidence-inspiring, approachable, predictable, accountable professional. In order to survive, she must know herself very well, have developed a sense of self-awareness, an intense sensitivity to the human condition and the capacity to look on her job as a challenge.

Exhibit 3-1. Institutional Prices—Fears—Prejudices—Expectations of Nursing Leadership

	The Board	Administration	Support Departments	Physicians	Staff in Dept. of Nursing
I. Those things they consider important **A.** Enlightened settings	• Reputation of the institution • Fiscal state of the institution	• Care is good, cost is reasonable. • Operation runs effectively.	• Responsiveness to service • Recognition of their importance to goals of institution	• Outcomes of care • Their authority and autonomy	• Patients • Patients' families • Accountability for practice • Colleague relationship with physicians
B. In unenlightened settings	• Control of staff in hospital • Consumer public	• No complaints from anyone • Cost is minimal	• Survival — "getting their oar in" (being heard)	• Power • Dow Jones averages	• Their economic welfare • Their status
II. Those things they fear **A.** Enlightened settings	• Damaged image of the institution • Fiscal failure	• Public • Impending insolvency • Government controls • Litigation	• The unexpected: "What will they do next?"	• Litigation • Amorphous, undefined loss of control • Governmental intervention	• Jeopardy for patients • Making a significant error
B. Unenlightened settings	• Takeover by physicians, administration • Confrontation with community	• Diminished "profits" • Interaction with patients • Confrontation with physicians	• The boss • Nursing department and power associated • Being uninformed	• Loss of power • Loss of income	• Wrath of physicians • Loss of what they consider a "power base"
III. Preconceived notions: **A.** Enlightened settings	• Doctors "get patients well." • Nurses merely make patients comfortable. • Nurse-administrators are necessary. • Quality care is patient-focused.	• Administrators are facilitators for caregivers (clinical staff). • Major decisions, including planning, require nursing input. • Nurse-administrators must be in top level management.	• Expectations of this department change regularly and with great frequency. • Patients are the most important focus of the institution.	• The authority of medicine is self-evident. • Quality patient care requires an interdisciplinary approach.	• Patient comes first! • Physicians are colleagues. • Nurse is advocate of patient and family. • Administrators are supportive of quality care.

	The Board	Administration	Support Departments	Physicians	Staff in Dept. of Nursing
B. In unenlightened setting	• It is unimportant to interface with nurse-administrator. • Physicians are most significant group in the institution. • Nurses are necessary but not particularly significant.	• Administrators are major decision makers in health care system, except for clinical issues. • Nurse-administrators may be unnecessary. The most you can hope for with regard to nursing is detente. • Nursing can be expected to take on any task whatsoever.	• Administration cannot be trusted. • Nursing is too powerful (ubiquitous) Doctors are the most important persons in the hospital (not patients).	• The hospital is the doctor's workshop. • Nursing in an arm of medicine and can be so represented. • Administrators power is misplaced.	• Doctors are all-powerful. • Patients **do not** "come first." • Administrators are not to be trusted.
IV. Expectations of nursing leadership A. Enlightened setting	• Accountability for nursing (Quality of care) and cost of that care. • **Availability**	• **Availability** • Accountability for department of nursing 1. Outcome of care 2. Cost of care 3. Staff to provide care • Participation in top level management • Nurse-administration will provide unique input to goals and operations.	• Effective communication • Collaboration • **Availability**	• Clinical and administrative competence • Collaboration • **Availability**	• Will represent nursing staff effectively • Will facilitate promotion of quality nursing care. • Is the advocate for the staff nurse • Can be trusted • **Availability**
B. In unenlightened setting	• Seen but not heard.	• Loyalty to administration • Keep the doctors happy • Maintains status quo set by administrative and medical staff • Minimal contact with board • Minimal communication with and expectation of administrative staff	• **Very little**	• Loyalty and attentiveness • Immediate responsiveness to physician • Submission • Control by physician group	• Attempt to control • Little advocacy • Little knowledge or appreciation of clinical nursing issues and problems

Nursing administrators must cultivate more than just skills. We must shape our own destiny, responding to a public whose presence is upon us. That public awaits a state of enlightenment about the role of nursing in the world of health care. Nursing leadership in every community must provide that enlightenment.

LEADERSHIP, LEARNING, AND CHANGING THE STATUS QUO

By Chris Argyris

Changes in the status quo involve leadership. Yet an examination of the current literature on leadership shows that most studies describe leadership activities as they exist and/or utilize criterion variables embedded in the present state of affairs. We need more research that illuminates how the present state of affairs can be changed and what role leadership can play in this quest.

Implicit in my position is the assumption that there may be something ineffective or dysfunctional in the current state of society. Donald Schon and I suggested that our society presently programs individuals with theories of action that generally are counterproductive to individual growth and organizational effectiveness. Moreover, these same theories are used to design organizations. One consequence is that even if applied effectively, they tend to create organizational stagnation or organizational deterioration. Knowledge is needed to suggest how we may break out of this self-sealing cycle that, as John Gardner has argued, could lead to a societal catastrophe.

Leadership has been defined as effective influence. In order to influence effectively, a leader requires on-line, repetitive learning about his influence. In order to solve ill-structured, complex problems, a leader also requires on-line, repetitive learning about how well substantive issues are being explored. Effective leadership and effective learning are intimately connected.

Studying about learning in terms of potent, real-life problems for which solutions are to be applied and tested in the noncontrived world means that the research methods to be chosen must meet certain criteria. They must not rule out the complexity of real life—or, if they do, they must specify precisely how the knowledge learned in the experimental setting can be used in the noncontrived world. They must involve their subjects easily and deeply so that they maintain their interest over long periods of time. They must not require keeping secret the design of the experiment from their subjects; indeed, they should permit their involvement without losing the power of making generalizations about human learning. They must be capable of eliciting behavior on the part of their subjects in such a way that the subjects cannot hold the design responsible for their actions. Otherwise, they may see no reason to accept personal responsibility for their behavior. The methods must be so powerful that the intended consequences can be brought about even under the most adverse circumstances, recognizing first, that their subjects may initially question their applicability and effectiveness (but not their moral validity); second, that their subjects are not able initially to behave in ways required by the experiment; third, that group behavior initially will be counterproductive; and last, that there will be few societal supports or rewards for learning the new behavior (otherwise we would be educating for the status quo).

I believe that it is possible to create these conditions in adult-learning environments with the requisite attracting, holding, and learning power.

THEORETICAL FOUNDATIONS: THEORIES OF ACTION, ESPOUSED THEORIES, AND THEORIES-IN-USE

We start with three key assumptions:

1. Human action is shaped by the theories of action held by people. Leading and learning are examples of shaped human action.

2. People hold two kinds of theories of action. First is the theory that they are aware of and report; this we call their **espoused** theory. Second is the theory they hold that can be determined by observing their behavior; this we call their **theory-in-use**.

3. Espoused theories vary widely. However, there appears to be very little variance among theories-in-use. To date, 95 percent of the variance may be included under one model—what we call Model I. The reason should become apparent as the research is described.

Picture human beings who have programmed themselves to behave in ways that are consistent with four governing values or variables (Exhibit 3-2). These are 1) to achieve the purpose as the individual has defined it; 2) to win, not lose; 3) to suppress negative feelings; and 4) to emphasize rationality. In any situation, human behavior represents the most satisfactory solution people can find consistent with their governing variables.

I have further hypothesized that human beings have also learned a set of behavioral strategies that complement their governing values or variables. The primary strategies are to control unilaterally the relevant environment and tasks and to protect themselves and others unilaterally. The underlying behavioral strategy is control over others. People vary tremendously in the way they control others, but few people do not behave in ways that control others and their environment.

These behavioral strategies, in turn, have consequences for the individual himself, for other people, and for the environment. Briefly, they tend to produce defensiveness and closedness in people because unilateral control does not tend to produce valid feedback. Moreover, unilaterally controlling behavior may be seen by others as signs of an individual's defensiveness.

In addition, I have hypothesized that these consequences tend to generate a particular kind and quality of learning that will go on within the individual and between the individual and the environment. There will be little public testing of ideas (especially those that may be important and threatening). Consequently, individuals will neither seek nor receive more than a modicum of feedback that genuinely confronts their actions. They will tend to play it safe; they are not going to violate their governing values and upset others, especially if the others have power. Moreover, whatever learning individuals acquire will tend to fall within the confines of what is acceptable. This is called single-loop learning because, like a thermostat, individuals learn only about those subjects within the confines of their program. They will find out how well they are

Exhibit 3-2. Model I

Governing Variables for Action	Action Strategies for the Individual and Toward His Environment	Consequences for the Individual and His Environment	Consequences for Learning	Effectiveness
Achieve purposes as the individual perceives them	Design and manage environment so that the individual is in control over the factors relevant to him	Individual is seen as defensive	Self-sealing	Decreased effectiveness
Maximize winning and minimize losing		Defensive interpersonal and group relationships	Single-loop learning	
Minimize eliciting negative feelings	Own and control task	Defensive norms	Little public testing of theories	
Be rational and minimize emotionality	Unilaterally protect self	Low freedom or choice, internal commitment, and risk taking		
	Unilaterally protect others from being hurt			

hitting their goal (maintaining a particular temperature). However, few people will confront the validity of the goal or the values implicit in the situation, just as a thermostat never questions its temperature setting. Such a confrontation would constitute double-loop learning. A teacher in a classroom, for example, may learn (single-loop) to ask students more specific questions in order to control student responses more readily; or the teacher may learn (double-loop) to reduce requirements for control in the classroom.

For most people there is a gap between their espoused theory and their theories-in-use, a gap of which they are unaware. Two reasons underlie this blindness: First, most people's theories-in-use include a proposition that states in effect, "If you see someone whose behavior is incongruent with what he or she espouses, for heaven's sake don't tell him or her because it will upset him or her and you will run the risk of eliciting

feelings of rejection and hostility.'' Second, people programmed with Model I theories-in-use are so busy controlling others in order to win, to advocate their position, and to do so in a way that cannot be disproved or publicly tested that they create self-sealing processes. The others, for their part, are so busy fighting back (they, too, are trying to win, advocate, and control) that there is little incentive for helping others to learn, especially if it may strengthen the others' position.

MODEL II AND
DOUBLE-LOOP LEARNING

One possible model has been recently suggested that would lead to consequences that are the opposite of Model I, a model identified by Schon and myself as Model II. The governing variables of Model II are valid information, free and informed choice, and internal commitment. The behavior required to satisfy these values is not the opposite of Model I. For example, Model I emphasizes that individuals be as articulate as possible about their purposes, goals, and so forth and simultaneously control others and the environment in order to assure achievement of their goals. Model II does not reject the need to be articulate and precise about one's purposes. However, it does reject the unilateral control that usually accompanies advocacy because the purpose of advocacy typically is to win. Model II couples articulateness and advocacy with an invitation to others to confront one's views and possibly to alter them in order to reach a position that is based on the most valid information possible and to

which everyone involved can become internally committed. This means the individual (in Model II) is skilled at inviting double-loop learning (Exhibit 3-3).

Each significant Model II action is evaluated in terms of the degree to which it helps the individuals involved generate valid and useful information (including relevant feelings), solve a problem in such a way that it remains solved, and do so without reducing the present level of problem-solving effectiveness.

The behavioral strategies of Model II involve sharing power with anyone who has competence and who is relevant in deciding or implementing an action. The definition of

Exhibit 3-3.   Model II

Governing Variables for Action	Action Strategies for the Individual and Toward His Environment	Consequences for the Individual and His Environment	Consequences for Learning	Effectiveness
Valid information	Situations or encounters are designed to enable participants to originate actions and experience high personal causation	Individual is experienced as minimally defensive	Disprovable process	Increased effectiveness
Free and informed choice			Double-loop learning	
Internal commitment to the choice and constant monitoring of the implementations		Minimally defensive interpersonal relations and group dynamics	Frequent public testing of theories	
	Task is controlled jointly	Learning-oriented norms		
	Protection of self is a joint enterprise and oriented toward growth	High freedom of choice, internal commitment, and risk taking		
	Protection of others is bilateral			

the task, the control over the environment, is shared with all the relevant participants. Saving face, one's own or the other person's, is rejected because it is seen as a defensive, nonlearning activity. If face-saving actions are necessary, they are planned jointly with the people involved.

Under these conditions, individuals will not tend to compete to make decisions for others, practice one-upmanship, and outshine others for the purposes of self-gratification. In a Model II world, people seek to find the most competent people to make a decision. They seek to build viable decision-making networks in which the major function of the group is to maximize the contributions of each member so that a synthesis, whenever it develops, is based on the widest possible exploration of views.

Last, under Model II conditions, if new concepts are created, the meaning given to them by the creator and the processes used in developing them are open to scrutiny by all who are expected to use them. Also, the creator feels responsible for presenting evaluations in ways that encourage others to confront them openly and constructively.

If the governing values and behavioral strategies just outlined are used, the degree of defensiveness within individuals, within groups, and among groups will tend to decrease. Free choice will tend to increase as will feelings of internal commitment. The consequences for learning should be an emphasis on double-loop learning that confronts the basic assumptions behind ideas or present views and that publicly tests hypotheses.

The end result should be increased decision-making or policy-making effectiveness, increased effectiveness in the monitoring of decisions and policies, and increased probability that errors and failures will be communicated openly and that participants in an action will learn from the feedback.

CASE OF THE NONPROFIT ADMINISTRATORS

So much for theory. Does it sound like a tall order? Is it clear that the switchover from a Model I to a Model II mode of behavior will take much time, involve much pain and agonized self-doubt, and require much professional assistance for the few with the motivation to run the course? All true—as our experience with a dozen different groups over the past several years has demonstrated. One study, research of managers in the governmental sector, illustrates the hypothesis tested in these dozen different learning environments. Knowing the models and having the opportunity to practice—under supportive conditions—may be a necessary, but is not a sufficient, condition for individuals to discover-invent-produce-generalize about the new Model II behavior.

The majority of the 100 manager-students were people with two to five years' experience as educational administrators, teachers, middle managers, governmental officials, middle- and top-level city and state officials, and a few first- and second-level business managers. All had read **Theory in Practice** [29] which described Models I and II in detail. The models were discussed in three two-hour class sessions. Toward the end of the sessions, the oral examinations that were held illustrated that the class members had mastered the key concepts in both models. Also, the students reported a strong interest in learning to behave in accordance with Model II.

At the beginning of the fourth session, the students were asked to read the following short case:

One of your subordinates has been performing inadequately for several months now. You've talked to him/her several times, and each time he/she has promised that performance would get better, but you don't see any evidence of this. Since you prefer not to fire him/her, you decide to make one more attempt. He/she walks into your office and asks: "Did you want to see me?"

They were asked to discover-invent-produce a solution. The production had to contain two parts, a short scenario of what the students as the actors in the case would say and do plus their feelings and thoughts about their behavior. They kept the original copy for a week as the basis for class discussion, and they gave the carbon copy to one of the faculty.

During the period between classes, the faculty members analyzed the cases to infer the degree to which they approximated Model I and Model II. All of the scorable cases (about 85) were categorized crudely in terms of the behavioral strategies manifested by the actors. Six behavorial strategies were identified:

1. The respondent attempts to get directly to the point that the subordinate is not producing adequately.

2. The respondent believes the subordinate is wrong but he wishes to start out indirectly and hopefully on a positive note.

3. The respondent couches the issue by asking if he (respondent) has a problem. ("Yes, come in, I want to talk about a problem that I have.")

4. The respondent begins by describing his feelings of discomfort, by attempting to place the subordinate at ease, and then by describing the problem with the subordinate's performance.

5. The respondent asserts that the subordinate has a problem, that the respondent is there to help and not to punish (not to fire).

6. The respondent asserts that both have problems and perhaps both can be of help to each other.

All these behavioral strategies approximated Model I. No matter how direct or indirect, how warm or how cool the interviews began, the respondents tended to approximate Model I theories-in-use. To illustrate how this judgment was arrived at, let us examine a scenario that illustrates the first of the behavioral strategies listed:

Respondent: (Hope this won't hurt his feelings too much.) Yes . . . I'm disturbed because I don't see much improvement.

Subordinate: I think my work has improved. I've had more work lately so that may be why you think there are more errors.

Respondent: (He doesn't really understand that there's a problem. That's a lie about more work. This is aggravating. I ought to just fire him, but actually he's kind of nice and comfortable to have around.) I don't agree that you've had more work to do. In any case, I simply can't go on seeing this kind of work. What do you think we ought to do?

Analyzing this scenario we find:

1. The respondent began by telling the subordinate he was disturbed because there had not been any improvement in his work (illustrates making judgments without publicly testing them).

2. The respondent's first feelings (the parenthetical inserts) illustrated an attempt to satisfy the Model I governing variables of minimizing the expression of negative feelings.

3. The respondent's reaction to the subordinate's comment was an assessment made of the other subordinate that was stated in such a way that it was not testable. Moreover, no attempt was made to test it publicly.

4. The covert assertion that the subordinate was lying was not tested publicly, partially in order not to arouse hostility.

5. The feelings of aggravation were suppressed (again minimizing the expression of negative feelings).

6. At this point, the respondent asserted that the organization could not be used to fulfill the subordinate's needs; the subordinate must perform. Yet the respondent, by being willing to keep the subordinate when he believed he or she should be fired, was fulfilling his personal needs in a way that may be inimicable to the organization's.

7. The first two sentences in the final voiced response showed the respondent's taking unilateral control. The last sentence appeared incongruent with unilateral control. The subordinate probably experienced it as the crucial question—namely, what he or she was going to do.

How typical are these responses? If we examine scenarios that are five to ten times longer than this, the pattern remains the same. That is, if the individuals begin with a Model I theory-in-use, they continue using the same theory-in-use. The changes that may be noted are that the dialogues become even more entrenched in Model I and the inconsistencies become more pronounced and glaring. The self-sealing processes become compounded and the level of holding back and/or deception increases. Moreover, these results continue when people use different modalities to express themselves (for example, going from writing to speaking to tape recording).

Subsequently, the manager-students broke down into small groups and studied the first strategy, chosen because it represented the most frequently used strategy. As consultants to the writer of the case, their task was to design an intervention to help the writer of the case cope with the problem in ways that approximated Model II. They were asked to invent a strategy and to appoint someone to produce the strategy.

After one-half hour of small group discussion, the class reassembled. The faculty member said that he would take the role of the writer. Each group representative described the intervention that they invented and then he/she would produce it through role playing.

The faculty member asked that the class monitor his behavior to make certain that he was not making it difficult for each group representative. The dialogues were all tape recorded. All of the inventions by the 11 small groups represented a mixture of Model I and Model II theories-in-use.

For example:

1. "He [the superior in the first case] should create an atmosphere where both can be open and share their feelings."

2. "He should create a situation so that each of them can develop the other's behavior rather than simply focus on her behavior."

3. "He should clarify for her the concrete expectations of work performance and the area that prevented him from firing her in spite of her inadequate performance."

4. "He should not control every aspect of the situation, including trying to minimize her expressing her negative feelings."

It appears that the students were learning Model II because they were inventing strategies that approximate Model II conditions. But such learning was at the conceptual level. What happens when the students attempt to transform the inventions (espoused theory) to theory-in-use?

We were able to obtain data to answer this question when the representatives from each group attempted to produce the inventions in the role-playing with the instructor. All the productions were judged by the class, the faculty members, **and the representatives who produced the inventions** (the latter after reflection), as approximating Model I. Moreover, an analysis of the transcript of the class discussion showed that when the productions were analyzed and discussed by the class members, these discussions also adhered to Model I.

Thus we have people who had read **Theory in Practice**; who had discussed it with one of the authors for three two-hour sessions; who met for a half hour to design the beginning of a Model II intervention; who invented Model I and Model II interventions, but who produced only Model I interventions. More-over, it was the members of the class who had identified the inventions and produc-tions as approximating Model I. Also, the class agreed that the faculty member could not be held responsible for the Model I behavior. Finally, an analysis of the mem-bers' behavior while they were commenting on the production of each group showed that these responses also approximated Model I.

It is important to keep in mind that no representatives were aware that, when they produced their group's solution, they had produced a Model I intervention. Nor were the students aware that they did the same thing when they tried to help the representa-tives become aware that they were not pro-ducing Model II interventions. Thus the class members could invent Model II solu-tions but were unaware that they could not produce them.

Looking back on these cases, we note that the students produced solutions that, the class concluded, illustrated Model I theories-in-use. For example: In the first example of an invention for the case quoted earlier, the respondent invented a solution that was to create an atmosphere of mutual inquiry, yet the respondent (and the class) judged the production to be the opposite. Attributions and evaluations were made about the re-spondent's behavior that were never tested. The attributions and evaluations were hid-den by the use of questions. The camouflage apparently worked only for the producer. Everyone else recognized the covert meanings.

In summary, motivation by itself is not the key to learning. As Don Schon and I ex-plained in **Theory in Practice**, the learning process is a cycle that involves 1) discovering the problem, 2) inventing a solution (concep-tual map), 3) producing the invention (per-forming in terms of actual behavior), and 4) generalizing what has been learned to other settings.

Each step in the cycle involves getting the participants to become aware of something of which they had habitually been un-aware—for example, the discrepancy be-tween their espoused theories and their theories-in-use.

People who wish to learn Model II theo-ries-in-use must re-educate themselves in each phase. They need to learn to discover-invent-produce-generalize about how to dis-cover, how to invent, how to produce, and how to generalize. Fortunately, people are not computers: they do not expect to be locked into their programs. They become in-creasingly frustrated, angry, and tense as evidence accumulates on their inability to help themselves or others to gain the com-petence they seek. Such feelings are a necessary part of the learning process. Learning that involves change in the govern-ing variables of a theory-in-use comes about only through dilemmas—through an indi-vidual's gradual realization that he is con-fronted with a progressively intolerable con-flict of central elements in his theory-in-use.

It is these reactions that lead people to become defensive—which, in turn, may lead people to use learning cycles that are protec-tive. These cycles themselves may increase the difficulties that created the frustration and anger in the first place. Hence we have self-sealing processes that create cumulative defensiveness in the actors involved. In the hands of competent faculty, however, it is these cumulative, self-sealing, defensive re-actions that can provide a breakthrough to learn Model II.

PRESIDENTS APPLY MODEL II

Another group consisting of six entre-preneurs, all presidents of their respective companies, is in the process of moving from Model I toward Model II. They have at-tended six sessions (ranging from two days to one week) over a period of three years.

After the presidents had successfully invented and produced Model II solutions in the classroom (a painful process similar to that undergone by the 100 administrators), they faced the big challenge—taking their solutions and experimenting with implementing them in their own companies.

Two problems were foremost in their minds. First, and the one to which they alluded throughout their sessions, was concern about the reaction of their subordinates when they began to exhibit their new leadership behavior. Second was discomfort about the prospect of behaving incompetently—as one man put it, "Making asses of ourselves in front of our people."

Turning to the first problem, the presidents had serious doubts that their subordinates would understand or see Model II behavior as relevant or practical. Because they themselves had expressed the same reactions toward Model II early on in their education, this lent credibility to their fears. Another, and probably more powerful, source of fear was the presidents' knowledge that, in their relationships with their vice-presidents, they had made many hidden assumptions, practiced many deceptions, and suppressed many doubts, all in the name of acting constructively toward them. For the presidents now to begin to behave in ways that they had previously rejected could arouse concern if not disbelief and bewilderment on the part of subordinates. And if this did happen, subordinates would probably withhold these feelings. This, in turn, would mean an increase in suppressed tension and/or an increase in overt discomfort on the part of subordinates. All these conditions would make introduction of Model II theories-in-use even more difficult.

To compound the problem, the presidents did not believe that they had mastered the new theory-in-use. Indeed, part of the process of mastering it required that they use it effectively in the "real" world. This greatly concerned the presidents because collectively their view of an effective president was one who was "strong." To be strong entailed behaving with confidence and approximating perfection. They believed that they could achieve neither criterion if they attempted Model II interventions at this time in their home settings.

The presidents began to experience several new dilemmas. On the one hand, after years of hard work within the seminars, they had begun to discover, invent, and produce new behavior and meanings that they valued. On the other hand, they feared experimenting with the new behavior back at home because of the negative reactions of their subordinates.

They had also learned in the seminars to handle such dilemmas by testing publicly the assumptions embedded in them. For example, their fears about negative reactions on the part of their subordinates required surfacing and testing. If they did not feel fully competent in behaving in accordance with Model II, they had learned to say so publicly. They had also learned to openly assert that what they were going to do was an experiment and that it might not be as successful as they had hoped.

Unfortunately, these cures made the illness worse. If they feared going public with their assumptions, testing these fears publicly would compound their fears; if they felt unsure about their new behavior, candidly saying so would make them appear weak in the eyes of their subordinates. To test this publicly would be embarrassing and bring to the surface their feelings of weakness—feelings that, in their minds, presidents should not express.

"I would not mind going through all this," said one president, "if I knew they wouldn't become confused and disorganized." A faculty member (one of my associates in the seminar) asked this president if he were willing to test that assumption publicly. "There you go again," he responded, "suggesting cures that make the problem worse."

The presidents realized that they were in a double bind. If they chose to experiment, they believed that they could be embarrassed and also harm the functioning of the top group. If they decided to withdraw, however, they would have to admit to themselves that they were controlled by fear and feelings of weakness. To be controlled by such fears obviously would be a sign of weakness, something they all found difficult to accept or admit.

This was a key moment in the group's learning process. Examining the transcript indicates that, although the diagnosis was painful, the choice to move ahead appeared natural and relatively simple. They decided that they had to be masters of their own fate; therefore, if the next step was to experiment, experiment they would.

The learning seminar became the base for the new operation. Each president chose a key issue—such as confrontation of an ineffective executive, development of an effective top-management problem-solving process, or reduction of an operating budget by 20 percent. They discussed it in detail and, with the help of others, invented a range of solutions. Each was produced by the president, with the other presidents acting as hard-nosed, disbelieving, confused, concerned subordinates.

After continual practice that helped them to discover, invent, produce, and generalize new interventions, the presidents began to feel confident enough to try their respective experiments in their own organizations. Several had designed experiments involving one or two persons. Several were interested in exploring Model II theories-in-use with their entire top group. Some experimented alone; others invited a faculty member. All tape-recorded their experiments or wrote

detailed scenarios that became a rich source of data for further learning. In all cases, the presidents experienced both success and failure. It was most interesting to see how easily they accepted their failures as episodes from which to learn and how willing they were to say so publicly. This, in turn, unfroze their subordinates and opened them up to explore their relationships not only with their superiors but also with each other and their own subordinates.

Not all subordinates liked Model II interventions (rare **or** well done). Some preferred the old ways of behaving and were frank enough to say so. Reading the transcripts, we saw that the presidents were attacked for behaving in ways that were perceived as weird, impolite, and potentially destructive of group cohesiveness. The fears the presidents had expressed were confirmed. However, the presidents did not become angry or punitive. They encouraged these expressions and, drawing from their seminar experience, used them to explore their impact as well as the foundations of cohesiveness within their groups. Perhaps one reason that the presidents could begin to deal with other people's fears effectively was that they had learned no longer to fear their own fears. Because they had begun to learn how to manage their own fears, they could use their newly acquired skills in helping others express and manage their fears.

Implications from the Six Entrepreneurs

At the most obvious but still meaningful level, there is the fact that the six entrepreneurs have made progress in experimenting with Model II in their own organizations, are making progress at the present time, and hopefully will make further progress in the future. That few people at the top would currently choose Model II as their preferred theory-in-use, that even fewer people are competent to make the changeover from Model I to Model II even with prolonged professional assistance, does not diminish the significance of what the six entrepreneurs have achieved so far. Only a few years ago, I wrote that "our own experience and the published research suggest that there now does not exist a top-management group so competent in meeting the requirements of the new ethic (the values incorporated in Model II) that they do not lose their competence under stress." I also expressed the belief that some groups and some organizations eventually would achieve that competence—a belief that our experience with the six entrepreneurs is in the process of confirming.

At another level, our experiences with the six entrepreneurs have deepened our knowledge of what is involved in learning to learn. This newly acquired knowledge, in turn, should enable us to help other groups similar to the six entrepreneurs in traveling the same road with a little less travail and pain.

What did we learn about learning? The adult learning processes with which we have experimented have turned out to be primarily cognitive. This does not mean that feelings did not surface. Indeed, the fear of fear and fear of embarrassment, hostility, failure, and so forth were continually experienced. However, the presidents coped with these feelings as components of their theory-in-use. Instead of asking, for example, why they feared failure, the participants learned to ask how they could test their fears and behave in ways that made them obsolete.

Following Model II theories-in-use, for example, the presidents did not choose to explore their personal histories to discover the roots of their fear of fear. A theory-of-action perspective informed them that the

way to cope with fear of fear was to create learning conditions with those people with whom they were presently involved—initially the other presidents in the seminar and eventually their own subordinates back home. As you may recall, this strategy created some problems, but it was facing these problems that led to progress. To repeat the sequences of action:

• They asked what, in the present context, operated as causes of their fear.

• After some discussion, they concluded that it was their fear that, if they behaved in an experimental, uncertain manner, their subordinates might become anxious because they wanted and expected strong leaders.

• Having made the conclusion explicit, they realized that it was, in effect, a series of assumptions about their respective subordinates. According to Model II, assumptions should be tested publicly before they become guides to action.

• This produced a double bind. Publicly to test these fears would compound their fears and probably upset their subordinates. To refuse to test publicly their attributions would mean that they withdrew from an action that made rational sense because they were afraid. To suppress rationality because of personal fears was to be weak.

• The presidents opted to experiment and learn. They utilized seminars to design their experiments, make many trial runs in front of each other (each simulating their worst fears), and develop confidence in their ability to respond effectively to expected resistance or confusion.

• Each president performed his experiment in his home setting differently, and each had varying degrees of success. However, each collected directly observable data, the Model II approach to testing concepts, and learned from his failures. Many subordinates reported surprise concerning the degree of openness of their superiors to explore their failures as well as design further experiments. Indeed, this openness to learning appeared to lead subordinates to explore some of the ineffectiveness among their own relationships.

• The competence to learn from failure and the way their subordinates rewarded their openness to learning served to raise the presidents' levels of aspiration for the next experiment and served as evidence that their fears were not based on valid information. As a result, their fears about experimenting in company settings began to diminish.

IMPLICATIONS FOR LEADERSHIP

Leadership theory will have to distinguish between results obtained at the level of the espoused theory and those at the level of the theory-in-use. To date, the preponderance of data employed in leadership research, including the data used by Professors Vroom and Fiedler, is at the espoused theory level. Research that remains at the espoused theory level runs the risk of missing 1) the incongruities between espoused theory and theory-in-use, 2) the blindness to these incongruities, and 3) the unawareness of the awareness that people have about their capacity to discover, invent, produce, and generalize theories of action that challenge the unchallengeable and question the unquestionable. If leadership education is ever to tackle core issues, these factors cannot be ignored.

To the extent that these factors are ignored, leadership education becomes a part of the existing theories-in-use. To the extent that this happens, leadership education will tend not to question the group, organizational, and societal factors that encourage Model I behavior. Leadership education becomes limited to education within the

status quo—education that, at best, may transform the world of espoused theories of action and yet have little or no impact on theories-in-use.

Leadership theory and theory about everyday life may overlap much more than has hitherto been assumed. Theories of action shape human behavior under all conditions, and theories-in-use are all minitheories of leadership in that they are theories of influencing others to increase one's own effectiveness. Our research suggests that even those who seek to be followers do so because that is their most effective way of gaining the level of control they seek over their personal lives.

Moreover, Model I theories-in-use are explicit leadership theories that focus on advocacy and unilateral control in order to win. These theories-in-use are consonant with those presently embedded in formal pyramidal structures and management theory. Indeed, this is probably no accident and requires much research.

Strong leaders in a Model I world may well be effective enough to control the world adequately to achieve organizational goals. Leaders whose strength is based on high advocacy and unilateral control over others also tend to hold attitudes that their subordinates need to be controlled, that they fear confronting people with power, that the competition among themselves is great, and that, if left to themselves, the group would fall apart. These assumptions are self-sealing because they are caused by the leadership style in the first place (or, if subordinates had these predispositions before the leader arrived, this style reconfirms and reinforces their utility).

One result of attributing fears and brittleness to one's subordinates is to make such attributions undiscussable because, as we saw in the example of our six entrepreneurs, such a discussion would be a cure that makes the illness worse. Granted, introducing Model II theories-in-use in organizations is fraught with potential failure and fear; but under Model II conditions, these possibilities must become discussable.

As our experiences with the six entrepreneurs have shown, it is possible over a period of years to change the theories-in-use of a group of company presidents from Model I to Model II, to create conditions in which their espoused theories and their theories-in-use are congruent, and to introduce Model II theories-in-use in the organization despite the fears and possibilities of failure. We can say about our six presidents (who in each case began as the quintessential Model I manager—"the kind of man I would never work for myself," as one self-description put it) that they had made the transition to being the kind of Model II manager who habitually practices double-loop learning. Once we can say that about the man at the top, the organization is on its way.

Many of the problems confronted and resolved under Model II conditions were serious problems that might never have been confronted at all under Model I or, had they been confronted, might have been less effectively resolved. One organization cut nearly 20 percent of its operating budget, with the entire top-management group participating in the process. In another case, the need for an executive position that the president believed the vice-presidents wanted was eliminated when, after a more open discussion, the presidents and the vice-presidents developed a new set of operating procedures that made the proposed executive vice-presidency unnecessary. The relationship between a chairman of the board (and owner of the company) with the president (whom the former had appointed personally) began to deteriorate because the latter's performance had not measured up to expectations. The problems were discussed openly and solutions were generated that pleased both men. More importantly, the resolution of the problem did not place the vice-presidents in the dilemma of having to take loyalty oaths toward the owner or the president. An unprofitable venture that the president hesitated to close down (because he had originally decided to create it) was cancelled with the help and advice of the vice-presidents, who had become more open with the president. Last, an organization faced up to the problem of what would happen when and if the president sold out—this being the kind of problem that probably never would surface in a Model I world.

Of course, we have made only a beginning. The presidents have taken the essential first steps in creating a Model II behavioral world with their immediate subordinates. In those instances in which subordinates responded positively, they, in turn, have taken the first painful steps toward creating a Model II behavioral world with their own subordinates. Actually, at this point most of the vice-presidents are where their bosses were three years ago. Relations among the vice-presidents and with the vice-presidents and their subordinates constitute an important inhibiting factor within these organizations.

Much remains to be done. We have said that the formal pyramidal structures that characterize most organizations are embodiments of a Model I theory-in-use. Before we can give an organization a Model II label, its structure, planning mechanisms, and policy-making procedures must all become congruent with Model II theories-in-use. And everyone within the organization, from the highest to the lowest, must understand, accept, and practice Model II as his or her theory-in-use.

All this will take years—and may never take place except in a relative handful of organizations. None of this detracts from the progress so far, progress worth recognizing, even celebrating, and worth advancing.

THE AMBIVALENCE OF ORGANIZATIONAL LEADERS: AN INTERPRETATIVE ESSAY

By Robert K. Merton

Reprinted with permission of the author from *The Contradictions of Leadership,* published by Appleton-Century-Crofts, 1970.

Consider the popular imagery of the leader in an organization. For some of the many below him in the hierarchy, he is secure, knowing, decisive, powerful, dynamic, threatening, driving, and altogether remote, acting in clear or obscure ways to affect the future of the organization he leads. At eye level, he is more often seen as filled with troubled doubts as he tries to deal with the ambivalences and contradictions of his status. And if his feet are made of a substance more solid than clay, it is because on his climb to the top and with the aid of those who help hold him there, he has learned to still the doubts, to live with the ambivalences, and to cope with the contradictions of his position.

The abundance of people—and if the leader leads, these must inevitably be called the (not necessarily passive) followers—are not altogether unaware of this complex situation. In the political arena, the daily manifestations of the ambivalences and contradictions which afflict the leader have attained the status of a sportive spectacle; periodically, box scores are presented in the press on the current standings of our eminent political figures as their public decisions delight some strata and alienate others. In other spheres of leadership, too, the con-tradictions of the position have become public victuals.

Although many ambivalences of leadership are common to all sorts of organizations—political and economic, religious and academic—this essay will deal primarily with that numerous company of American leaders, the topmost business executives, known, ever since the days of Thorstein Veblen, as captains of industry.

Whether it is an organization for business or another purpose, there are only two routes to the top: one from within, the other from without. Each has its particular advantages and handicaps; each produces its own syndrome of ambivalence.

The leader coming from within the organization will tend to know it well: its signal strengths and weaknesses, its style of management and the quality of its managers, its living history and its aspirations, its markets, products and prospects. But perhaps he will know it too well. Friendships and personality clashes have much the same tendency to induce myopia in a leader. And corporate associations of long standing, except in the case of the most detached and widely experienced of managers, have a way of limiting the leader's horizons, of impairing his vision, of restricting his view of

145

possibilities for the future. What has stood the organization in relatively good stead in the past—in terms of organizational goals and of the methods deployed to move toward them—may continue to be carried on. This may be good enough for the immediate if not the longer-run future. But the very value of his intimate knowledge of the past successes of the organization may induce what Veblen unforgettably described as a "trained incapacity": a state of affairs in which one's abilities come to function as inadequacies. Recurrent actions based upon training, skills, and experiences which have been successfully applied in the past result in inappropriate responses **under changed conditions.** As the leader from within adopts organizational measures in keeping with his past experience and employs them under new conditions which are not recognized as **significantly** different, the very soundness of training for the past may lead to maladaptation in the present. In Burke's almost echolalic phrase: "People may be fit by being fit in an unfit fitness." Their past successes incapacitate them for future ones.

The assumed advantages and handicaps of the in-route to the top are typically reversed with the leader coming from outside the organization. He does not know the company in depth. Practically all of his first months, if not years, will be spent in its study—its past performance gauged against its past potentials, the capabilities of its people, material resources, aggregate aspirations. The organization must endure a period of contemplative inaction. But if his lack of firsthand acquaintance with the organization is a defect, it also has its qualities. He brings few built-in biases toward the particular organization and its parts (although he will, of course, inevitably have his own collection of biases grown outside). But having no emotional involvement with the past of the organization, he is—or the more easily can be—capable of opening himself to all kinds of innovative possibilities. He can more readily perceive ideas which may have been floating around the organization for years. He brings, surely, a fresh—not necessarily, a correct—approach to the problems and opportunities of the organization he now leads, and an expertise gained outside the intellectual confinement inherent in every organization. Still, he brings with him from outside no guarantee of success.

The ambivalences of organizational leadership begin, then, at the beginning. They are found in the route the leader followed to get there, whether from within or from without. They begin with the sum total of his previous organizational experience and with the interaction of his own capability for adaptive growth and all the foibles and creative impulses of the organization he leads.

Regardless of his origin, the newly made leader of the organization soon confronts another ambivalent situation. As leader, it is his obligation to bring to his position a vision of the future, a sense of direction as to where he wants the organization to go. He must obey the further organizational imperative, on pain of failure, of sharing his private vision with the total organization. For vision that is remote from the values and wants of the many around him becomes transformed into self-defeating fantasy. Within these obligations are planted the seeds of several conflicts and ambivalences.

The more sharply the leader defines his vision, the more confident he is of his own role (and vice versa). But in sharpening his vision he has narrowed his options. And in narrowing his options he has limited the number and kind of his subordinates who will, with enthusiasm, perceive and work toward the goals encompassed in that vision. For people who are to release their energies toward the attainment of goals must have a voice and a hand in shaping those goals. They must, in short, have a sense of some mastery over their own destinies. Yet with each slice of power released by the leader—and it is power, i.e., the ability to make something happen, which, in the final analysis and however broadly defined, is the core of leadership—the greater becomes his own condition of uncertainty.

A second kind of conflict is in the offing between the leader who projects his own vision and the organization itself. The more "different" and the more radical that vision happens to be, the greater will be the conflict. For just as the leader comes to his position as the synergistic sum of his experiences, so too he leads an organization which is the synergistic sum of **its** experiences. Indeed, the experiences of the organization will be more deeply ingrained—through its history, traditions, culture, and the sheer inertial structure of all organizational life—than those of any of its individual members. Under such conditions, flexibility in the executive grip may, with only seeming paradox, produce a steadier hand.

Whether his vision is large or small, the leader will want—indeed, will have an emotional need—to shape the organization, to change it, to mold it into a creation which, at least in part, he can claim as his own. Yet, inexorably, he in turn will be shaped, probably without his recognition, by the organization, by its needs, its capabilities, its standards. At some distant time, should he look back, he will be unable to distinguish between the changes he has wrought and the ones which have been wrought in him.

Another ambivalence confronting the leader is built into the circumstance that although nothing succeeds like success, in organizations increments of success become self-limiting. This means for the leader that the organization will be at one and the same time a continuing source of great pleasure and acute pain. The leader will demand that the organization improve its performance,

raise its standards, increase its efficiency. And when, through the objective measurement of the budget or some other device, improvement is discovered and entered into the corporate record, the leader will take great pleasure in it. But to obtain even a tittle of improvement, the leader will find that he must pass through a prolonged period of anguish, during which he feels (and sometimes is) personally responsible for the outcome and, in any case, is held accountable for it. And he will find, too, that unlike an individual who is able to assimilate and use new information for sometimes spectacular improvements in performance, a complex organization functions, for the most part, on precisely the reverse principle: that, after a certain point, as organizational efficiency improves, further improvement becomes increasingly difficult.

Still another ambivalent requirement exacted of the leader calls for him to have pride in his organization, to induce or reinforce the pride of other members of the organization, and still to keep the extent of that collective pride in check. The leader must somehow arrange for that composite of pride that is justified by accomplishment and commitment but, at the same time, he must recognize that pride can become overweening, no longer sustained by continuing accomplishment. This is often expressed in what Theodore Caplow has designated as the "aggrandizement effect": "the upward distortion of an organization's prestige by its own members." Having studied 33 different types of organizations—among them, banks and Skid Row missions, department stores and university departments—he found that members overestimated the prestige of their own organization (as seen by outsiders) eight times as often as they underestimated it. Sooner or later, contact with the world of reality forces the prideful leader and his followers to discover that both utilitarian and moral assets waste away if they are not energetically renewed and extended. For the rest of the social system will not stand still. And so organizations which would move with it must continue to engage in both innovative and adaptive change.

While the leader is concerned, perhaps above all else, with pulling the entire organization to higher levels of performance, he will often be put in the contradictory position of being unable to meet the demands for facilities to provide superior performance by the organization's individual parts. He is presented with a classical dilemma of organizational decision. Deeply committed to the goals of the organization, two or more separate departments are each doing their utmost to serve the best interests of the total organization by maximizing their distinctive kinds of contribution to it. But, often, even typically, maximizing the contribution of one part means limiting the contributions of other parts. There is, in the striving for organizational excellence—although many hesitate to concede it—a balance to be struck that means curbing the single-minded drive for maximum performance by the component parts. The dilemma of decision can be transcended only by having the distinct parts rise to a concern for the whole. Commitment to the goals of the organization then takes precedence over commitment to the goals of the department.

From his relations to his subordinates emerge a variety of other dilemmas, ambivalences, and contradictions for the organizational leader. It is the manager's responsibility, perhaps his very first responsibility, to sustain the people who report to him. He is, in fact as well as in word, "the first assistant of his subordinates." Yet who is to sustain the leader? Granting that topmost leadership is "the loneliest position on earth"—a bit of excusable hyperbole—it is not necessarily so for most organizational leadership; not, that is, under the proper circumstances. Those circumstances have to do, of course, with the kind of support that the subordinates give to their superior in his position of leadership. Turned half-circle and viewed from the position of leadership, this means the degree of confidence which the leader has in each of his subordinates.

There is, in every superior-subordinate relationship, a complex of interactions. At the root of them all, when they are effective interactions, is the confidence or trust that each has in the other. In organizational life, the prime ingredient of reciprocal confidence is not competence alone, although the importance of competent performance of roles should not be underrated. It is the first stone on which confidence is built.

This reminds us that leadership is not so much an attribute of individuals as it is a social transaction between leader and led, a kind of social exchange. And again, though some leaders sense this intuitively, the rest of us must learn it more laboriously. Leaders assist their associates in achieving personal goals by contributing to organizational goals. In exchange, they receive the basic coin of effective leadership: trust, confidence, and respect. You need not be loved to be an effective leader, but you must be respected.

Identifiable social processes produce the respect required for effective leadership. First, respect expressed **by** the leader breeds respect **for** the leader. As he exhibits a concern for the dignity of others in the organizational system and for their shared values and norms, he finds it reciprocated. Second, as has been said, he demonstrates technical competence in performing his own roles. He does not merely talk about competence, he exhibits it. Third, the effective leader is in continuing touch with the germane particulars of what is going on in the human organization. For this, it helps, of course, to be located at strategic nodes in the network of communication that comprise much of every organization. But structural location is not enough. Once situated there, he provides with calculated awareness for two-way communication. He not only lets the other fellow get an occasional word in edgewise; he lets him get a good number of words in straightaway. And the effective leader listens: both to what is said and to what is not said in so many words but is only implied. He allows for both negative and positive feedback. Negative feedback, as a cue to the possibility that, in his plans and actions, he has moved beyond the zone of acceptability for his colleagues and subordinates; positive feedback, as a cue that he has support for his initiating actions.

Fourth—and on this accounting, finally—although the leader in a position of authority has access to the power that coerces, he makes use of that power only sparingly. He gives up little and gains much in employing self-restraint in the exercise of his power. For once he has gained the respect of associates, it is they, rather than the leader directly, who work to ensure compliance among the rest of their peers. Leaders only deplete their authority by an excess of use, and that excess is not long coming when leaders, having lost the respect of their subordinates, anxiously try to impose their will. Group experiments in sociology have found that the more often group leaders use the coercive power granted them, the more apt are they to be displaced. The experiments confirm what has long been thought; at its most effective, leadership is sustained by noblesse oblige, the obligation for generosity of behavior by those enjoying rank and power. Force is an ultimate resource that maintains itself by being seldom employed.

In a word, what instills confidence between superior and subordinate is joint commitment: commitment to one another and to agreed-upon organizational goals. It is this mutual commitment which encourages even the leader who is temperamentally inclined to retain the reins of power in his own hands to delegate not only responsibility but also authority to his subordinates, which allows him to rely more on corporate consensus than on authoritarianism in the making of decisions, and which, in turn, motivates the subordinate to request (or through muted symbolism, to demand) the exercise of responsibility and power commensurate with his position rather than to suffer in silence the close-handed intransigence of the oligarchic leader.

This train of thought need not be pursued very far in order to identify what has been emerging as one of the major contradictions facing modern organizations, including, as a prime special case, business organizations. This contradiction is found in the tendencies working simultaneously toward democratic rule and the more traditional authoritarian rule. This is something far deeper and more fundamental than a matter of the relationship between two or more individuals or even groups of individuals. It not only affects the style of management, the relationship between organizational units, the definition and operation of management, but touches upon the very purpose of the organization itself.

In recent years, behavioral scientists—notably such organizational investigators and theorists as McGregor, Herzberg, Argyris, Likert, Lawrence, and, in his own way, Peter Drucker—have shown to a growing number of corporate executives that efficiency and productivity lie in the direction of a more democratic or participative management. This proposition can be overstated and it often has been. Nevertheless, there is now a growing abundance of evidence testifying that **under certain conditions** democratic leadership is the more efficient in making for productivity of products **and** of valued human by-products.

All the same, styles of leadership continue

to vary. The repertoire of styles is extensive; and, it would seem, only few leaders have or acquire the versatility to shift from one to another style as changing circumstances require. There is the authoritarian style, in which the leader is insistent, dominating, and apparently self-assured. With or without intent, he creates fear and then meets the regressive needs of his subordinates generated by that fear. He keeps himself firmly at the center of attention and manages to keep communication among the others in the system to a minimum. Ready to use coercion at the slightest intimation of divergence from his definitions of the situation, the authoritarian may be effective for a while in times of crisis when the organizational system is in a state of disarray. But, particularly for organizations in a democratically toned society, extreme and enforced dependence upon the leader means that the organizational system is especially liable to instability.

The democratic style of leadership, in contrast, is more responsive. It provides for extended participation of others, with policies more often emerging out of interaction between leader and led. It provides for the care and feeding of the self-esteem of members of the system, but not in that counterfeit style of spreading lavish flattery on all and sundry egos in the vicinity, after the fashion once advocated by the merchants of interpersonal relations who would have us make pseudofriends by inauthentic expressions of sentimentality. (Remember G. K. Chesterton's finely wrought distinction: "Sentiment is jam on your bread; sentimentality, jam all over your face.") The democratic style of leadership does not call for indiscriminate and unyielding faith in your fellow man; some people are **not** to be trusted or respected or supported in their incompetence and willful malevolence. What the democratic style does call for is the introduction and maintenance of systems of relations which make for a grounded trust in others and for the human by-product of enabling people in the system to actualize their capacities for effective and responsible action and so to experience both authentic social relations and personal growth, each giving support to the other.

Precisely because one is committed to the ideal of democracy, one must be mindful of countertendencies in organizational systems. To begin with, there is a tendency toward what the German sociologist, Robert Michels, as long ago as 1915, excessively described as "the iron law of oligarchy." He was led to this "law" through which new organized minorities acquire dominion within organizations by examining the case of democratic organization. He found there the seeming paradox that leaders initially committed to democratic values abandoned those values as their attention turned increasingly to maintaining the organization and especially their own place within it. The danger is plain. Leaders long established are often the last to perceive their own transition toward oligarchy, toward a form of control in which power is increasingly confined to the successively few. And leaders long established are apt to confuse the legitimacy of their rule with themselves.

The Michels brand of organizational pessimism poses grave problems for the business leader who would be both competitive and compassionate. The temper of the age suggests, however, the necessity of developing a response that utilizes a countervailing force to Michels' iron law. Such a force finds expression in the rule of thumb which says that the solution to the deficiencies of democracy is more democracy.

A particular ailment of organizational leadership was long since diagnosed by Chester Barnard as "the dilemma of the time lag." In this phrase he referred to the problem of discrepancy between organizational requirements for immediate adaptive action and the slow process of obtaining democratic approval of it. This is an authentic dilemma, not easily resolved. Democratically organized groups can cope with it only by having their members come to recognize **in advance** that, remote as they are from the firing line of daily decision, there will be occasions in which decisive action must be taken before it can be fully explored and validated by the membership. To earn the right for leases of independent decision, democratic leaders must provide for continuing accountability. They must be accountable not only in terms of the criteria they themselves propose but in terms of the often more extensive criteria adopted by other members of their organization and by the wider society.

This brings us straight to another ambivalence and dilemma confronting the organizational leader. One of the traditional responsibilities of the corporate leader, no less than the political one, and the cause of many contradictions in which the corporate executive is involved, is the need to balance the interests of groups which have a legitimate (and sometimes not so apparently legitimate) call on the resources of the organization.

The most obvious interest in the business corporation is economic and the most obvious interest groups are composed of employees, owners, and consumers. Striking a balance among these three groups alone—to say nothing here about the needs of increased capitalization, of the local community, and of the society beyond—poses basic contradictions of thought and action. In the one sphere of employee interests, for example, the business leader is often torn by the question of whether he should seek to attract labor at minimum cost or whether he should ensure for the organization a pool of quality labor by paying top dollar; whether he should place more or less emphasis on fringe benefits as opposed to wages and

salaries; whether he should ensure security of employment to the possible short-term detriment of the corporation or whether he should seek maximum efficiency (which means, to put it bluntly, staff layoffs during periods of lax activity) to the possible long-term detriment of the coporation. Such questions are not completely resolved in the marketplace. The decisions turn more nearly on the system of values within which the corporation functions. These values, in turn, are imposed not so much by the economic function of the corporation as by its culture, traditions, history of recent experience, and by the personal proclivities of its leaders within the current context of the polity, the economy, and the society.

In this same sphere of employee interests, but now in a wider sense, the corporate leader must balance or arbitrate a secondary and often equally important interest: what is to be the share of the corporate resources allocated to each unit? What percentage of the budget will be allotted to manufacturing, research and development, advertising, computerization, the development of staff, and so on? It is a tempting belief that such questions are resolved in the organizational hierarchy solely by considerations of corporate need based on objective analysis and authoritative projections. But this is seldom the case. The business leader is as much circumscribed as the political leader by "political" constraints internal to the organization. And with all the accounting systems of planning, programming, and budgeting now in force and yet to come, one suspects that this will continue.

All this takes us back to the structural and functional aspects of the position of organizational leader. He is, of course and above all else, a maker of decisions; not, be it noted, **the** decision maker. He differs from all the other makers of decision in the organization he leads in this: His decisions are ordinarily more consequential for the fate of that organization and for those parts of its environment affected by the ramified results of those decisions. He faces with fearsome regularity the need to assess conflicting interests, conflicting sentiments, and conflicting convictions within the organization. In this regard, there can be no rest for the sometimes weary leader. He is structurally located at the very node of conflicting wants and demands within the organization. His role requires him to acknowledge and work on these conflicts, not to deny them or to cover them over with the rhetoric of feigned consensus. He has the task of alerting the others to the sources of the conflict, to define and redefine the situation for them, to have them acknowledge in turn that decisions gauged in the light of the organization as a whole must often override the particular concerns of its parts.

It is no easy matter to discover what is in the best interest of the total organization, and so there is ample leeway for continuing disagreement. A degree of indeterminacy requires the exercise of reasonably confident judgment rather than the demonstration of certain outcomes. The leader may err in his calculated decisions engaging the conflicting interests and beliefs of his constituency. That is bad enough. But his greatest error comes in trying to evade these conflicts. Nothing catches up with an organizational leader so much as a conscientious policy of evasion which seeks the appearance of peace and quiet by avoiding decisions that might alienate this or that sector of the constituency. And **because** of a degree of indeterminacy about the validity of the decision, it is not merely the substance of his decisions that is consequential for the organization but the mode through which he arrives at them and the mode in which he makes them known. Effective leaders arbitrate and mediate the inevitable conflicts within the organization in such fashion that most of the members involved in his decisions feel most of the time that justice has been done. It is the role of the leader to act for the whole while interpreting for the parts. And so it is that even a substantively mistaken decision—as the limiting case—taken in ways that win the respect of associates and presented in ways that enlist their however reluctant assent will be less damaging than decisions which are substantively sound at the time but which have little support in the organization because they are taken as arbitrary and inequitable. The reason for this is plain enough. Organizational decisions become transformed into organizational realities only to the extent that they engage the willing support of those who must translate them into day-by-day practice. Without such support, the **initially** sound decision has a way of becoming converted into a subsequently unsound one.

Just as the corporate leader must balance the interests of interest groups within his organization, so he is caught in the even more difficult dilemma of balancing the interests of interest groups outside his organization. The direct relation between the portions of economic wealth distributed by the corporation to its various primary "publics" is reasonably well understood. Should dividends greatly increase, there will be less under static conditions for distribution to the workers in the form of wages and to consumers in the form of stable or lower prices. But conditions are not static; indeed, it is one of the important functions of the private sector to see to it—through innovation, cost control, new efficiencies—that they never become static.

The rise of consumerism can be ascribed, at least in part, to a growing public which, surfeited with material possessions, now demands that these same possessions be imbued with qualities which are not only economically profitable but socially desirable. Thus, in our autos we demand seat belts rather than chrome strips; in our drugs, efficacy rather than palliatives (or worse); in our health care, adequacy for all rather than for the few. In like fashion, the call for "relevance" and "meaning" in work cannot be ascribed only to the altogether alienated few but must be recognized as also representing the deepest drives for self-actualization and self-esteem among those who, already employed, have found a measure of economic security.

The leader of a significant business corporation must be both a "local" and a "cosmopolitan." By a local, I mean one who is largely oriented to his organization or immediate community which dominates his interests, concerns, and values. By a cosmopolitan, I mean one who is oriented toward the larger social world beyond his immediate organization or community, with extended interests, concerns, and values. The effective leader faces the task of combining both orientations and developing capabilities appropriate for putting both into practice. He must be able to look inward at his organization and outward at its concentric zones of environment.

And still the question remains: How shall the leaders of organizations steer their course through the ambivalences and contradictions of leadership? What concepts shall they use as their guide? Written by a man who has known throughout his adult life the pleasures and pains of leadership, the speeches in this book may be instructive.

LEADERSHIP FOR THE FUTURE

By Marjorie Beyers

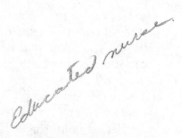

Leaders in nursing, like leaders in any other field, are purported to have a perspective of the past, the present, and the future. Experienced leaders may be said to have an advantage over newly emerging leaders because they have lived through the past. Their experiences not only give them the benefit of knowing how organizations and professions change over time—10, 15, 30, or 40 years—but also give them self-knowledge about how they can best function in their leadership roles to achieve change and personal satisfaction in the practice of nursing.

Newly emerging leaders may be said to have equal advantage over experienced leaders in that they are not fettered by past experiences. They also have the benefit of current education with knowledge of the most recent concepts and theories in their field, newly learned and freshly viewed. The newly emerging leaders may benefit from their lack of experience in that they have not yet become encumbered with such attitudes as, "I tried that in 1957 and it didn't work." As these leaders venture into their new and as yet "untried" functions, they have the advantage of the energy generated by their spirit of discovery and their sense of potential growth in the profession.

In this essay I explore some aspects of the past, the present, and the future to illustrate the current nursing leader's roles of leadership in organizations. I assume that professional nurses in organizations are working toward increasingly professional practice and that this practice takes place mostly in organizations. The relationship of the leader and of the professional to the organization is therefore an important focal point in the study of nursing leadership—one that can serve as a basis for sharing between experienced and novice leaders, a sharing that maximizes the advantages of each group for the benefit of the profession's growth.

Nursing leaders who hold positions of authority in organizations are concerned with achieving productivity in the organization—that productivity is patient care. Drucker writes that "to make the worker 'achieve' demands that managers look upon labor as a resource rather than a problem, a cost, or an enemy to be cowed. It demands that managers accept responsibility for making human strengths effective. And this means a drastic shift from personnel management to leadership of people." [30] This passage illustrates one of the problems of nursing leaders in organizations. They are shifting from "management functions" to leadership functions. Part of the reason for the magnitude of this shift in organizations is that nurses are emphasizing their own professionalism in current practice.

The shift toward professionalism in

nursing away from former task orientation of nursing practices in health care agencies is not unique to nursing. Drucker writes, "The most rapidly growing group in any organization, especially in today's business enterprise, are people who are in management, in the sense of being responsible for contribution to and results of the enterprise . . . The most rapidly growing group in business enterprise today are individual professional contributors of all kinds who work by themselves . . . and yet have impact on the company's wealth-producing capacity, the direction of its business, and its performance" [31]. This change, Drucker writes, results in problems with the structure and for the manager. He views the change as requiring solutions to problems; one of the major problems that ensues is that of communication. The professional in the organization has knowledge and expertise that are effective in achieving results for the entire organization. In this knowledge and expertise, the nursing professional becomes a leader. In Drucker's thesis, the manager guides the professional, interprets the professional's knowledge and functions into organizational terms, and serves as a channel for directing the professional's knowledge and expertise. Leadership in knowledge and expertise, according to Drucker, remains the professional's responsibility. The professional, in his view, is the teacher or educator of the manager.

Drucker's points are pertinent to nurses who are employed by health care organizations. Nurses are the "experts" in nursing care. Their expertise must be interpreted in the organization, channeled into the total input of the organization, and must contribute to the effectiveness of the organization. The organization must provide the support systems necessary to accomplish professional nursing effectively. When these conditions are not met, nurses run the risk of reverting to the mechanistic tasks of giving medications, ambulating patients, or giving treatments, the expected functional or task-oriented nursing roles of the past. These components of patient care can easily be emphasized in "mechanistic" organizations because they are more visible, more easily counted, and more controllable than some of the other components of holistic patient care. Do you agree that holistic care is the cornerstone of current professional practice in nursing? Do you agree that nurses have not yet achieved the provision of holistic patient care in most health care agencies?

The leader in nursing who is familiar with the past can better understand the nature of the change that nurses are endeavoring to bring about in health care agencies. All nursing leaders, whether they are experienced or new to the field are influenced by this past. It is helpful to understand that the current status of nursing is closely related to the current status of organizations in general. Like that of an individual, the current status of an organization is a product of, among other things, past experiences. A brief review of the evolution of management theories illustrates this point.

Consider, for example, that in the last half of the nineteenth century theorists began to define how organizations work. Frederick Taylor, known as the father of scientific management, was a student of management in this era. Through research methodology he studied ways to analyze jobs or tasks to improve productivity of employees. His beliefs were based in an approach to management that emphasized orderly progression of tasks to achieve productivity and training employees to perform the tasks correctly and effectively. In many ways, Taylor's approach to management is similar to the precepts of competency-based education used in many educational systems throughout the United States today.

Another theorist well known to students of management is Henri Fayol, who stressed planning and control in his management theories although he was concerned with management as a set of processes not limited to planning. The language of short-range and long-range planning can be traced to Fayol's writings. His perception of planning has endured and continues to be used in current management.

Yet another famous management theorist from the early days of management science is Max Weber. His contribution to management theory is most predominantly cited as his description of organizations as bureaucratic. Weber characterized effective organizations in a bureaucratic model that emphasized specialization of function, hierarchy of control, and impersonal relationships among employees. The purpose of the organization was to organize people to effectively and efficiently produce work. These organizational characteristics can be found in present-day hospitals. There are specialized departments and delineation of employees in a hierarchy of positions with authority flowing downward from the board of trustees, to the chief executive officer, to the nursing leadership personnel. Nursing professionals have been working to change some of these hierarchical relationships by recognizing the expertise of professionals to make decisions. They have been endeavoring to incorporate nurse specialists, such as nurse clinicians, into traditional organizational structures. Nurses have also been working to change the concept that impersonal relationships are more effective than appropriate open expression of emotions and feelings among nurses and between nurses and patients. This trend is illustrated in nursing literature; in the forties, for example, remaining objective, detached, and uninvolved was accepted behavior for nurses. The literature of the sixties is replete with articles about recognition of social processes and the need to deal openly with feelings, expressing them appropriately in

patient care, and learning to recognize the human components of nurse–patient interactions. Current nursing literature contains increasingly more substantive information about the basis for understanding emotions and feelings and about concepts of behavior to be incorporated into care planning.

This brief description of early management as guided by the scientific approach and the trend to emphasize human relations in management serves to illustrate the transition in expected leadership behaviors in organizations that has been ongoing for many years. This transition is described to some extent in the evolution of leadership theories included in Luthans' essay in Unit 1. The change from authoritative (bureaucratic or scientific) to participative management (human relations) is the underlying theme in many of the leadership theories. Findings of the Ohio State Studies, McGregor's Theory X, Theory Y, and Likert's System Four Management theory emphasize participative management in accordance with changes in organizational theory toward emphasis on human relations. Because management is closely related to expectations of leaders in organizations, changes in management theory imply changes in expected leadership behaviors. The leader in an organization may be constrained by the organization's postulates about management, particularly if the leader focuses on participative management in an organizational structure that is highly bureaucratic.

Warren Bennis has dealt with concepts of organizations of the future in his writings. He believes that core tasks confronting organizations of the future can be categorized in five major areas. These are integration, social influence, collaboration, adaptation, and revitalization [32]. The problems in the task of integration are those of integrating the individual with the organization. Bennis writes, "It is the ratio between individual needs and organizational demands that creates the transaction most satisfactory to both'' [33]. In this context, the nurse must achieve satisfaction from performance of his or her profession in the organization while at the same time, the organizational goals must be met. The organization must provide incentives, the professional must be motivated, and the rewards to each must be balanced.

Social influence, in Bennis' terms is the task that refers to use of power in organizations. Hierarchical structures of bureaucratic organizations tend to centralize power in one or a few persons. This centralization of power in a few conflicts with current-day "professionalism" in nursing in which the nurse has expert power to perform and expects that the organization will not only permit but respect that power.

The third core categorical task presented by Bennis is collaboration. He cites dysfunctional intergroup conflict as the problem to be overcome in expanding organizations where there is fragmentation and division of groups. He writes, "Modern organizations abound with pseudospecies, bands of specialists held together by the illusion of a unique identity and with a tendency to view other pseudospecies with suspicion and mistrust [34]. In order to counteract the resulting conflict, Bennis suggests that real conflict should be used to generate productivity and creativity and that pseudoconflict should be minimized. The nurse–doctor conflict so frequently mentioned is an example of two pseudospecies that are often involved in pseudoconflict. Can you think of other pseudoconflicts—or real conflicts?

Adaptation, the fourth core task, is cited by Bennis as being related to uncertainty and rapid change in the environment. Nurses in hospitals are dealing with rapidly changing events, expansion of knowledge and technology, and increasing stress. Although patient care cannot be routinized even in the most bureaucratic organizations of the past

or present, the tendency to use routines to provide stability and to increase productivity of workers is less useful in today's health care organizations than it formerly was to establish the basis for nursing practice productivity. It is fair to state that the care environment is undergoing rapid change in today's health care organizations. In order to accommodate patient needs in this changing environment, there must be sufficient numbers of nursing professionals who have the expertise to make decisions required to give effective care.

The last task, revitalization, is perhaps the most challenging to the leader. Bennis writes that elements of revitalization are:

> An ability to learn from experience and to codify, store, and retrieve the relevant knowledge.
> An ability to "learn how to learn," that is, to develop methodologies for improving the learning process.
> An ability to acquire and use feedback mechanisms on performance, to develop a "process orientation," in short, to be self-analytical.
> An ability to direct one's own destiny. [35]

The leader who fits Zaleznik's description of leadership, presented in Unit 2, is the one who revitalizes organizations. This is the type of leader who will shape the future of nursing. How will this leader bring about the future goals and directives of the profession?

First of all, the leader must recognize that there is unlimited potential for the development of nursing in the future health care industry. In the introduction to *Primary Care: Where Medicine Fails,* it is written, "Why can't American medicine live up to its wondrous potential. Here the 31 participants including the four authors agree that the U.S. needs a better system for the delivery of health services. No apparatus exists to define and ensure basic primary care services. But while prescriptions for the ills of the medical care system are easy to make, these experts acknowledge that the complexity of making the needs of future patients compatible with those of health providers is almost over-whelming" [36]. From this passage it is clear that no one knows how to shape the future—it seems fitting that nurses as one of the largest groups of health care providers are capable of taking up this challenge to their leadership. The power of nursing knowledge and expertise for shaping improved health care in the future is great, if nurses in the aggregate can acknowledge and use this power.

Nurses tend to be other-directed. It is acceptable to be concerned with and to direct energy to patients. Nurses are less comfortable being concerned about and directing energy toward themselves. In order to use their power of knowledge and expertise effectively in the health care system however, nurses must accept being concerned about themselves as well as about patients. Earlier it was assumed that nurses would like to provide holistic nursing care. Gadow writes about some of the problems in delivery of holistic nursing care and she questions, "to what extent is the whole person of the healer—in this case the nurse—a necessary corollary for optimal healing of the whole patient. . . . The issue requires a sound and new conceptual framework within which to develop means for unifying and transcending the once contradictory relation between professional and personal" [37].

Nurses as a group are not unique in attempting to integrate the personal with professional involvement. As demonstrated by many of the leadership theories presented in this anthology and by an earlier description of the transition in management from the scientific to the human relations approach to dealing with people, this integration is a goal of many different types of professionals. Nurses, as products of their society, have problems and concerns that are similar to those of other groups in that society. Recognition that the goal of integration is a common one in the society should make

nurses aware of the fact that they have the same resources within their world as do other groups. Nurses, particularly nurse-leaders, should take advantage of the opportunities that exist to deal with their problems in achieving integration. In so doing, nurses should work with others who are seeking the same goals in different fields, and should present themselves as collaborators in this endeavor.

Integration of the personal and of the professional as suggested by Gadow is part of the process of integrating professionals with the organization. Bennis cites this type of integration as one of the core tasks of leadership for the future. How should the professional nurse become a part of health care organizations? This is a question that leaders of the future must deal with head-on. In answering this question the leader will have to deal with basic organizational structures, changing them to accommodate professional practice that is congruent with organizational goals. Nurses will have to deal with the essence of the professional practice. They will have to decide what nurses ought to be doing in providing patient care. Analysis of patient care needs and of the input of other professional groups in meeting these needs is important in determining the essence of nursing practice and concomitant nursing functions. Nurses then have to determine what types of resources and support systems they will need to provide this nursing care of the future. The resources and support systems may exist in present-day health care organizations or the organizations may have to be adapted or changed, and new resources and support systems may have to be developed. In this era of economic constraint, nursing leaders are challenged to determine how the available resources should be organized and developed to provide care for the future. New systems may be formulated through reordering, revitalizing, or restructuring the existing ones.

Human resources are essential in the health care industry. It is to determine the best uses of one group of these human resources, nurses, that the profession should direct its attention in development of the profession's future. If nurses were to realize and make use of the social power inherent in their membership, the profession in general could exert increasing influence on the health care industry. Even though nurses do not earn the most money when compared to other health care professionals and even though they tend to be employed rather than in independent practice, the size of the nursing group as compared to other health professions is a source of social power. Nurses may be encumbered in achieving social power by their history, by the norms and beliefs they hold about nursing and that are held by society. If nurses wish to change the norms and standards of nursing practice they must realize that other systems may also have to change; social influences of one group usually affect other related groups.

Bennis emphasizes power when discussing social influences. In attaining social power, nurses should pay attention to the responses they make to "society" and to others in the health care industry. Ginzberg writes that "One important mechanism that can facilitate a society's adjustment to change is its sense of timing and appropriateness of response. One of the dangers facing a dynamic society, especially one that has shed its inhibitions to experiment, is the tendency to venture too much, too quickly. There is also the opposite danger that it will move too slowly or with too little force when new departures are called for" [38]. To develop a sense of timing and appropriateness of response, it is necessary that nurses increasingly work toward development of the profession within the structures of society so that they are attuned to behaviors or changes that are needed and that can be accepted by the public as well as by nurses.

It is interesting to speculate that nurses will have to resolve their feelings of alienation to more perfectly become attuned to societal changes. Alienated persons tend to be inner-directed, and this concern with self can function to limit reception of stimuli from external sources. Alienation is a common sociological phenomenon that occurs in all types of groups. Hall develops the thesis that workers feel alienated when they experience powerlessness, meaninglessness, isolation, or self-estrangement [39]. Many nurses feel that they have no power in their positions within the health care industry. In their perception administrators or more generally "organizations" wield power over them and they have no control or voice in the administration or organization. Do you know nurses who feel powerless?

Some nurses also feel that their positions are meaningless. The nurse who wishes to give holistic care and who consistently performs only daily assignments such as giving treatments or passing medications may feel that the position is meaningless in relation to that nurse's expectations for giving patient care. Nurses who attempt to bring about change and whose efforts are consistently resisted may also develop a feeling that their work is meaningless. What factors could be changed in nursing practice and in organizations to make nursing positions meaningful for all nurses? Is your position meaningful—is the work you perform meaningful to you?

Isolation occurs when people fail to develop supportive relationships in their jobs. It could be speculated that nurses who are attempting to make decisions and whose efforts are thwarted in so doing may feel isolated within organizations. Have you experienced this type of isolation? Are you able to express your opinions and ideas in the place where you are employed? Are your decisions recognized and used? And do your efforts make a difference in the quality of patient care? A common type of isolation expressed by nurses occurs in nurse–physician relationships. The nurses who perceive that the doctors make all decisions without benefit of nursing input may feel isolated from patient care management. There are many other sources of isolation in organizations, and many of them stem from perceived or real lack of power on the part of the person who develops feelings of alienation.

The last of the components of alienation, self-estrangement, is described by Hall as a sense of being detached personally from the work. If the work is perceived by the person as meaningless, if the person perceives that he or she has no power to make decisions or to use initiative, and if the person feels isolated within the organization, it is probable that the person retains the employment for purposes other than satisfaction with work performed. Hall writes that this person does not have a sense of pride in the work and views it as a means to an end. Do you know nurses who work, giving patient care, only because they want to buy a new car or renovate their homes or take an extended trip? The challenge to leaders is to deal with alienation in making nursing positions meaningful for nurses. It is the leader's function to accept that alienation exists in all segments of society and that causes for alienation can be discovered and dealt with constructively. Leaders must also avoid becoming consumed by feelings of alienation themselves—feelings which might result in their becoming detached and therefore would cause their demise as leaders.

One way to avoid feelings of alienation is for leaders to develop constructive support systems. Developing relationships with others in an organization is one way to establish these support systems. Developing relationships or alliances is cited by Kanter to be a source for accumulation of organizational power as well. Kanter writes, "More often neglected in the study of the accumula-

tion of organizational power is the importance of strong peer alliances, . . ." In Kanter's study it was found that peer alliances worked in several ways; through exchange of favors or information or through bargaining or trade. She found that people in organizations perceived that the group members needed one another and that leaders had developed a sense of helpfulness and sharing with their peers. The leaders were other-directed, not me-directed [40].

Peer alliance implies collaboration, one of the core tasks cited by Bennis to be accomplished by future leaders. Developing peer alliances in interdisciplinary networks could be one way that nurses can accumulate organizational power. This power should not be perceived as domination or as winning or losing. Instead, it should be perceived as power to collaborate on some equal ground. Bennis developed the theme that intergroup conflict could be dysfunctional. In his terms, pseudospecies and pseudoconflict can lead to this dysfunction. The problem that nurse-leaders of the future have is to determine which species are real and which are pseudospecies, which conflicts are real and which are pseudoconflicts, not important or relevant to the situation.

To develop the sense of real and of "pseudo," nurses must develop realistic concepts of nurses' capabilities, of how organizations function, how health professionals can collaborate, of the needs of patients, and of trends in society. The nurse who has formulated these realistic concepts can better differentiate between the real and the unimportant. It can be speculated however that what is unimportant or "pseudo" may be relative to different groups and to different situations; what is real in one situation may be unimportant in another. This speculation is grounded in the situational theories of leadership effectiveness described in Unit 1.

Organizational control, for example, is a

necessity and a reality in that it frees people to accomplish their work. How organizations are controlled may be relative to the particular situation or organization. To elaborate, rules are part of the process of organizational control. That rules are necessary is real; the type of rule used in a given situation or organization may not be "real" but instead may be termed a pseudorule (to take liberty with Bennis' terminology). The rule that is "real" is needed in the situation; the one that is unnecessary can create pseudoconflict. Formerly, for example, nurses working in hospitals were subject to the rule that they must wear caps. Recently, nurses have demonstrated that they can function effectively without wearing caps. One can then question, is the rule that nurses wear caps necessary or not? In some situations or in some organizations this rule may be necessary and as important as the rule that prescribes that nurses check the patient's identity before giving medication. The content of the rule is based in an established rationale that is important or necessary to effective functioning in a specific situation. Given the variations in organizations, what is real and what is unimportant may be relative to the organization.

While wearing or not wearing caps may not illustrate the essence of nursing practice, this example does illustrate that if nurses are to become better integrated with an organization, they must respond not only to their professional values and functions in the organization, but also to the situations and values pertinent to the total organization. Both nurses and organizations are challenged to adapt to changes. The current practice of not wearing caps in some organizations can be used as an example of adaptation by nurses. Nurses who do not find wearing caps necessary are adapting to societal changes in modes of dress, to changes in values about uniforms, and in some respects to the increased comfort with professional roles that are more dependent on knowledge and expertise than on external appearances. Have organizations in which nurses no longer wear caps made adaptations to accommodate the new mode of dress?

Like alienation, the need for adaptation is not unique to nurses, but is a common need of people in society who are experiencing the effects of a rapidly changing environment. How do individuals and groups deal with this rapid change? To discuss the change process is beyond the scope of this essay. Suffice it to say that nurse-leaders in the future can learn to use necessary change to their advantage.

How can change be used to the profession's advantage? To illustrate this point consider the idea that bureaucratic organizational structures may have to be changed to accommodate newly emerging nursing functions. Bureaucratic organizations tend to perpetuate themselves and to be resistant to change, but it is inevitable that health care organizations will change in accordance with new demands and new restraints. Nurses in this health care organization environment can recognize that changing structure is inevitable and can develop a rational thesis for the changed structure that supports emerging nursing functions. In order to obtain support of others in this organization it is important that nurses select relevant components of their practice and support systems in formulating the thesis for structural changes in the organization. The nurse-leaders of the future will increasingly have to be aware that what is real and what is "pseudo" may be different for their profession and for the organization. To resolve this potential conflict, these nurses must retain a clear vision of the mission of the nursing profession, patient care, in formulating plans for change. The substance of patient care is the commonality basic to integration of health professionals with health care organizations. Dealing directly and realistically with this substance facilitates communication among these professionals. For this reason, adaptation, or dealing with change, should be based in substantive theory or in educated intuition about patient care if the nursing profession's growth is to be accepted by other "educated" health professionals and managers in an organization.

Growth in organizations is of concern to those who administer them. What constitutes growth in an organization is speculative; growth is not always perceived as becoming bigger; it can also mean becoming better. Organizations can become better in quality of services, in scope of services, or in any other aspect that creative and resourceful leaders can devise for growth. The points listed earlier from Bennis' article outline some cogent ways to revitalize organizations or people or processes. Nursing professionals are increasingly becoming aware of the need to codify, to store, and to retrieve data. It is not sufficient to have data, however, it is also necessary to determine how to apply these data to devising nursing input for organizational growth.

It seems that revitalization can only take place if the other four tasks are also taking place. Integration, social influences, collaboration, adaptation—all of these tasks may lead to revitalization. To accomplish these tasks, development of consulting skills will be beneficial to nurses in leadership roles. Lippitt and Lippitt, in writing about the consulting process, outline decision-making areas in the process. These include diagnosis of problems and a concomitant framework of criteria and values for determining interventions, an orientation to collaboration, capacity to take risks, an orientation to identification of resources and to their appropriate use, and the ability to decide what interventions are appropriate given the best timing and methodology for the context [41].

In consulting one learns, and learning to learn is one of the tasks cited by Bennis to be important for future leaders. Argyris wrote about double-loop learning—the need to maintain or to create open systems for interchange, for obtaining feedback, and for participative communication. Using the consulting process in leadership supports his concept of double-loop learning. Leaders must also be cognizant of the need to continue to learn through both formal and informal methods. Attending conferences, classes, completing projects, participating in committees, and any other type of activity that necessitates study and exploration of new ideas and concepts are important in maintaining leadership capabilities. Another interesting method for learning that benefits both established and newly emerging leaders is use of the mentor system. Either being a mentor for another or having a mentor can also encourage development of the spirit of self-destiny.

The use of mentors for "bringing up" novices in a field is not unique to nursing. This method has been used in industry and in other professional fields for development of leaders. An advantage of this system is that it perpetuates the positive qualities of leadership; the benefit of experience, of accumulated knowledge, of self-knowledge, and of proven effectiveness for the novice who learns from the mentor. An effective relationship between student and mentor frees the student to become a leader by developing leadership talents with the support of the expert. The mentor may find that the student eventually surpasses his or her accomplishments—this may be expected when the student "solos" and performs in a world different from that experienced by the mentor. This different world results from changes in the times, from changes in the environment, and changes in the work to be accomplished. The novice leader's effectiveness is nurtured by the mentor to achieve destiny in future professional growth that stems from past accomplishments.

In Bennis' terms, achieving destiny is the

ability to control the future. In all of the actions that leaders take to influence the future, the selection of new leaders is crucial.

Maslow offers a solution to leadership selection. First, he created the perfect situation, (the eupsychian situation). In this situation leadership tasks were determined by the group or by the requirements of the objective, situation, or problem. The selected leader was the person whose qualifications met the task requirements and who identified with the task "so strongly that you couldn't define his real self without including that task." Maslow described the person as one who loves his or her work, is absorbed in it, and who enjoys the work—one who "can hardly think of himself apart from it" [42]. This leader, wrote Maslow, "Can be defined as the one who can get the job done best or who at least can help to organize things in such a fashion that the job gets done best" [43]. His description fits the person with an integrated personality who can integrate his or her functions with that of an organization. This is the leader that Maslow states has the "ability to take pleasure in the growth and self-actualization of other people" [44]. Perhaps this is the best type of leader for nursing because the future of the profession may be best assured if all its members experience growth and self-actualization.

FILLING IN THE MATRIX: LEADERSHIP IN ORGANIZATIONS

The third unit has integrated the theories presented in Unit 1 with the leader behaviors discussed in Unit 2. Decision making, use of power, and negotiation are three main themes in the selections included in this unit.

1. Focus your attention now on the methods you use when functioning as a leader in the place where you work, as they relate to our model.

   a. Select one major decision you have made within the past month and describe the process you used in making that decision.

      i. Did you make the decision alone? With others?
     ii. What sources of information did you use in making the decision?
    iii. What resource persons within and outside of the organization did you consult in making the decision?
    iv. Who and what was affected by the decision?
     v. What are the outcomes of the decision? (Is the matter finished? Did the decision open up new areas for discussion and decision making? Did you deal with reactions of others to the decision?)

   b. As you think about decision making in your leadership role, are some decisions you make based on personal preferences? Are others based on organizational preferences?

      i. Differentiate between decisions that are made on the basis of personal preference and those made on the basis of organizational preferences.
     ii. Do your work-related decisions differ from your home-and-family related decisions? From your professional-organization related decisions?
    iii. What processes do you use in making decisons with those you lead? Do you find yourself frequently vetoing decisions made by others?

2. Growth of professionals in an organization is a common concern in institutions such as hospitals that employ large numbers of knowledge workers. How the leader uses power may be directly related to the level of stimulation of professional growth in nurses you lead.

a. Consider how you use power in relation to the following power bases presented in this unit's content. Try to remember situations in which you used each power base and, for each situation, think of how your use of power affected the people involved in the situation and how they responded to your use of power.

  i. Reward power
  ii. Coercive power
  iii. Legitimate power
  iv. Referent power
  v. Expert power

b. How does the use of power by others in the organization affect you? How do you respond when:

  i. The president uses coercive power with you?
  ii. A clinical specialist in your department uses expert power with you?
  iii. Reward power is used by the board of trustees in a situation for which you are predominantly responsible?
  iv. The chief of medicine uses legitimate power in a patient care matter involving you?
  v. A peer department head from another discipline uses referent power with you?

3. Nurses are instrumental parts in a health care agency and the leader integrates the components of our model to accomplish patient care through the functions or actions of the nurses. One aspect of nursing leadership is to establish in the organization that "functions or actions" of nurses are professional endeavors. Consider your perceptions of this aspect of leadership.

a. Do you have a different set of ideals and goals for nursing in the organization than does the administrative staff? Than the physicians? The majority of the nurses? If not, what did you do to establish congruence? If so, what are you doing to "close the gap" to achieve congruence in ideals and goals? Examine the following possible approaches in relation to your behavioral motivation and approach to change:

  i. It is safer to maintain the status quo.
  ii. It is best to confront the physicians and administrators.
  iii. Persons from other departments should be involved in nursing organizational decision making.
  iv. Perceptions about nursing in the organization should be changed through subtle means.
  v. Professional organization membership is useful in dealing with nursing ideals and goals in the workplace.
  vi. Organizational requisites in the workplace are placing professional nurses in conflict with professional alliances.

vii. *Tradition has formed perceptions of nursing functions and actions in the organization.*

b. *You represent nurses and nursing functions and actions in many important departmental decisions. Using the content in Argyris's article, consider how you obtain the information used to formulate your presentations of nursing goals, needs, and plans to decision-making groups in the organization.*

i. *What techniques and methods do you use to obtain information about the status of patient care given by nurses in the organization?*

ii. *When you receive information from a variety of sources, which do you place most emphasis on in making decisions about nursing? Information from:*
   •*A group of staff nurses_____*
   •*A group of supervisors or coordinators_____*
   •*A group of physicians_____*
   •*The administrator(s)_____*

iii. *How do you sift the information you receive to prepare your presentations of nursing to the organizational administration? Do you feel well informed about nursing in the organization?*

iv. *Do those you lead feel supported by your actions in organizational decision making?*

c. *When serving as a member on a departmental level committee do you feel most comfortable making decisions that:*

i. *Are accepted by the majority of persons on the committee?*
ii. *Reflect the organization's goals?*
iii. *Are congruous with professional nursing goals?*
iv. *Represent the wishes and desires of nurses in the department for improving patient care from their perspective?*

It is anticipated that you will say "yes" to all of the above. What do you do (and how do you feel) when the decisions are the opposite of those listed above? Of the possibilities given, which is most applicable to your situation?

d. *Negotiation is a process in which a leader mediates between two forces or among many forces. Reflect on a situation in which you recently negotiated an agreement in light of the following:*

i. *What persons were involved?*
ii. *Is this situation representative of the concerns you most frequently negotiate?*
iii. *Was the outcome of your negotiation compromise? Consensus? Agreement to disagree?*
iv. *Is this outcome typical of your negotiation efforts?*

4. Leadership can be satisfying, but it also has elements of frustration. Consider how you deal with situations, the source of your rewards and of your frustrations.

    a. In your organization, is there a pattern of rewards for certain types of behavior?

        i. Rate the following types of behavior from 1 to 5, with 1 going to behavior you would most likely reward.
        ___ *Efficient* ___ *Moral* ___ *Professional* ___ *Economical* ___ *Loyal*
        ii. Do you think that the pattern of rewards in the organization is the same as your own pattern of rewarding behaviors in those you lead? How are they the same or different?

    b. Select the passages of Merton's article that are of most direct relevance to you. Do you feel ambivalent about your leadership? What type of support system do you use to maintain your perspective?

    c. Compare your perspective of leadership now with that you held when you first began working in the position you now have.

        i. Has your perspective of leadership changed?
        ii. Would you like to become a different type of leader than you now perceive yourself to be?
        iii. What would you like to do to continue to grow in your leadership abilities? What would you need to do?
        iv. What advice would you give to those who aspire to become leaders in nursing?

REFERENCES AND NOTES

1. Barnard, C. I. **The Functions of the Executive.** Cambridge, Mass.: Harvard University Press, 1974.
2. Greer, L. Professional self-regulation in the public interest: the intellectual politics of PSRO. In Proceedings: Conference on Professional Self-Regulation. DHEW Publication No. (HRA) 77-621. U.S. Department of Health, Education, and Welfare, June, 1975.
3. Levine, E., and Elliott, J. E. Analysis and Planning for Improved Distribution of Nursing Personnel and Services. Prepared for ANA Convention '76, June 4, 1976, Atlantic City, N. J.
4. Barnard, C. I., 1974.
5. Greer, L., 1975.
6. Levine, E., and Elliott, J. E., 1976.
7. Chaney, W. H., and Beech, T. R. **The Union Epidemic.** Germantown, Md.: Aspen, 1976, p. 125.
8. Colner, A. N. The impact of state government rate setting on hospital management. **Health Care Management Rev.,** 2(1), Winter, 1977.
9. Epstein, R. L., and Manson, L. A. First questions on the HEW handicap regulations. **Hospitals,** 51:19, 1977.
10. Maslow, A. **Eupsychian Management.** Homewood, Ill.: Irwin-Dorsey, 1965.
11. Bullough, B. Influences on role expansion. **Am. J. Nurs.,** 76(9), 1976.
12. Claus, K. E., and Bailey, J. T. **Power and Influence in Health Care.** St. Louis: Mosby, 1971.
13. Levine, E., and Elliott, J. E., 1976.
14. Jelinek, R. C., and Dennis, L. C. A Review and Evaluation of Nursing Productivity. In A Conceptual Framework for Nursing Productivity. DHEW Publication No. (HRA) 77-15. U.S. Department of Health, Education, and Welfare, November, 1976.
15. Marram, G., et al. **Cost-Effectiveness of Primary and Team Nursing.** Wakefield, Mass.: Nursing Resources (formerly Contemporary Publishing), 1976.
16. American Nurses' Association. Facts about Nursing. Kansas City. ANA, 1974.
17. Johnson, W. L. Educational preparation for nursing—1975. **Nurs. Outlook,** 25(9), 1977.
18. Sultz, H. A., Zielezny, M., and Kinyon, L. Longitudinal Study of Nurse Practitioners, Phase I. DHEW Publication No. (HRA) 76-43. U.S. Department of Health, Education, and Welfare, Bethesda, Md., March, 1976.
19. Strauss, A. **Negotiations: Varieties, Contexts, Processes, and Social Order.** San Francisco: Jossey Bass, 1978, Introduction.
20. Maslow, A., 1965, p. 39.
21. Burns, J. M., **Leadership.** New York: Harper & Row, 1978, p. 78.
22. Bennis, W. The Problem: Integrating the Organization and the Individual. In Monahan, W. G. (Ed.) **Theoretical Dimensions of Educational Administration.** New York: Macmillan, 1975, pp. 332-336.
23. Hicks, H. G., and Gullett, C. R. **Organizations: Theory and Behavior.** New York: McGraw-Hill, 1975, p. 238.
24. French, J. R. P., Jr., and Raven, B. The Bases of Social Power. In Cartwright, D. (Ed.) **Studies in Social Power.** Ann Arbor, Mich.: Institute for Social Research, 1959.
25. Schopler, J. Social Power. In Berkowitz, L. (Ed.) **Advances in Experimental Social Psychology,** vol. 2. New York: Academic Press, 1965, pp. 177-218.
26. Bachman, J. G., Bowers, D. G., and Marcus, P. M. Bases of Supervisory Power: A Comparative Study in Five Organizational Settings. In Tannenbaum, A. S. (Ed.) **Control in Organizations.** New York: McGraw-Hill, 1968, p. 236.
27. Bachman, J. G., Bowers, D. G., and Marcus, P. M. 1968, p. 41.
28. Berle, A. A., **Power.** New York: Harcourt, Brace and World, 1969, p. 37.
29. Argyris, C., and Schon, D. **Theory in Practice.**

30. Drucker, P. F. **Management Tasks, Responsibilities, Practices.** New York: Harper & Row, 1973. p. 304.
31. Drucker, P. F., 1973, p. 391.
32. Bennis, W. The Problem: Integrating the Organization and the Individual. In Monahan, W. G. (Ed.) **Theoretical Dimensions of Educational Administration.** New York: Macmillan, 1975, pp. 333–336.
33. Bennis, W., 1975, p. 333.
34. Bennis, W., 1975, p. 334.
35. Bennis, W., 1975, p. 336.
36. Andreopoulos, S. (Ed.) **Primary Care: Where Medicine Fails.** New York: Wiley, 1974, p. 3.
37. Gadow, S. Nursing and the Humanities: an Approach to Humanistic Issues in Health Care. In Bandman, E. L. and Bandman, B. (Eds.) **Bioethics and Human Rights.** Boston: Little, Brown, 1978, p. 310.
38. Ginzberg, E. **The Human Economy.** New York: McGraw-Hill, 1976, p. 59.
39. Hall, R. H. **Occupations and the Social Structure.** (2nd ed.) Englewood Cliffs, N. J.: Prentice-Hall, 1975, pp. 54, 55.
40. Kanter, R. M. **Men and Women of the Corporation.** New York: Basic Books, Inc., 1977, pp. 184, 185.
41. Lippitt, G. and Lippitt, R. **The Consulting Process in Action.** La Jolla, Calif.: University Associates, 1978, pp. 46–47.
42. Maslow, A. **Eupsychian Management.** Homewood, Ill.: Irwin-Dorsey, 1965, p. 122.
43. Maslow, A., 1965, p. 128.
44. Maslow, A., 1965, p. 131.

BIBLIOGRAPHY

Bauer, J. C. A nursing care price index. **Am. J. Nurs.,** 77(7), 1977.

Deloughery, G. L. **History and Trends in Professional Nursing** (8th ed.) St. Louis: Mosby, 1977.

Miller, M. H., and Flynn, B. C. **Current Perspectives in Nursing: Social Issues and Trends.** St. Louis: Mosby, 1977.

Miller, M. H. Academic inbreeding in nursing. **Nurs. Outlook.** 25(3), 1977.

Safier, G. **Contemporary American Leaders in Nursing.** New York: McGraw-Hill, 1977.

definition.
Styles - 31 - 33

Mental Health - leadership - 45 - 47
confidence - ed. gine - 89
fear - 91, 92, 96
maslow. - 94
Personality traits in leader. - 95.
nurses as leaders - 110 - 107.

CONTRIBUTING AUTHORS

Steven H. Appelbaum, Ph.D.

Associate Professor of Management
Faculty of Commerce and Administration
Concordia University
Montreal, Quebec, Canada

Chris Argyris, Ph.D.

James Bryant Conant Professor of
Education and Organizational Behavior
Harvard University Graduate School of
Education
Cambridge, Massachusetts

Chester I. Barnard†

Peter F. Drucker, Ph.D.

Clarke Professor of Social Science and
Management
Claremont Graduate School
Claremont, California

Carol Grangaard Heimann, R.N., M.A.

Night Relief Supervisor
St. Mary Hospital
Manhattan, Kansas*

Norman Hill, M.A.

Training Specialist
Exxon Company, U.S.A.
Houston, Texas

---

*This information reflects the author's position when the selection included in this anthology
was originally published.
†No biographical information available.

Fred Luthans†

Robert K. Merton, Ph.D.   University Professor
                                           Columbia University
                                           New York, New York

William C. Parrish, M.S.   Assistant Administrator
                                           The Deaconess Hospital
                                           Cincinnati, Ohio

Leo Plaszczynski, Jr., R.N.   Director, Nursing Service
                                           Candler General Hospital
                                           Savannah, Georgia

                                           (At the time the method described in the arti-
                                           cle was developed, the author was Director,
                                           Nursing Services, Burnham City Hospital,
                                           Champaign, Illinois)

June Werner, R.N., M.S., M.S.N.   Chairman, Department of Nursing
                                           Evanston Hospital
                                           Evanston, Illinois

Abraham Zaleznik, Ph.D.   Cahners-Rabb Professor of Social
                                           Psychology of Management
                                           Harvard University Graduate School of
                                           Business Administration
                                           Boston, Massachusetts

Index